More Praise for

THE PEGAN DIET

"Read this book right now to learn how to use food as medicine. Dr. Mark Hyman has the rare ability to show you how to eat in order to feel better while also fixing our food system from the ground up!"

—Dave Asprey, author of *The Bulletproof Diet*

"Dr. Hyman has done it again. By framing food as medicine, *The Pegan Diet* takes an innovative and important approach to wellness. This prescription will not only help prevent disease, it also has the real potential to dramatically reduce health care costs by getting to the root cause of disease."

—Congressman Tim Ryan

D0126762

THE
PEGAN
DIET

21 PRACTICAL PRINCIPLES FOR RECLAIMING YOUR HEALTH IN A NUTRITIONALLY CONFUSING WORLD

Mark Hyman, MD

Little, Brown Spark
New York Boston London

Copyright © 2021 by Hyman Enterprises, LLC

Little, Brown Spark
Hachette Book Group
1290 Avenue of the Americas, New York, NY 10104
littlebrownspark.com

First Edition: February 2021

Little, Brown Spark is an imprint of Little, Brown and Company, a division of Hachette Book Group, Inc. The Little, Brown Spark name and logo are trademarks of Hachette Book Group, Inc.

The publisher is not responsible for websites (or their content) that are not owned by the publisher.

The Hachette Speakers Bureau provides a wide range of authors for speaking events. To find out more, go to hachettespeakersbureau.com or call (866) 376-6591.

Illustrations by Courtney McNary

Printing 1, 2020

ISBN 978-0-316-53708-7 (hardcover) / 978-0-316-54178-7 (large print)
LCCN 2020946031

LSC-C

Printed in the United States of America

To the confused eater committed to better human and planetary health

Contents

THE
PEGAN
DIET

Introduction

Do we really need another diet book? No. Despite the title, the Pegan Diet is an un-diet—a simple set of principles blending science and common sense into guidelines promoting health, weight loss, and longevity that can easily be adapted to any philosophical or cultural preferences. What do we know about food? How do we know it? What conclusions can we draw from the data? How do we combine that with dietary, philosophical, social, and cultural preferences? As a physician on the front lines of the epidemic of chronic disease and obesity (one who has used food as the primary medicine in treating disease and optimization of health for 30 years), I am saddened by the diet wars and fad diets. Politics, religion, and nutrition are all equally polarizing.

The Pegan Diet started off as a joke. Years ago I sat on a nutrition panel at a conference between two friends—one doctor a Paleo proponent, and the other a vegan cardiologist. They argued vigorously for their points of view. To break the tension, I quipped, "Well, if you are Paleo and you are vegan, then I must be Pegan." Thus it all began. As I started to think more deeply about what I had said as a joke, I realized that most dietary philosophies, including Paleo and vegan, had far more in common with one another than most people realize, and far, far more in common with one another than with the Standard American Diet, otherwise known as the SAD diet.

In fact, Paleo and vegan camps (if we stick to the best in both approaches) are identical except for one thing: where to get protein. Animal products or beans and grains? That's it. Of course, you can be a chips and soda vegan, or a bacon and no veggies Paleo eater, but the best whole food expressions of each are so similar. Both promote a plant-rich whole foods diet; a diet low in starch and sugar, processed food, additives, hormones, antibiotics, GMOs; and, except for a small group of extreme low-fat vegan fans, a diet rich in good fats. They both even eschew dairy. And all the other dietary approaches—vegetarian, keto, time-restricted eating, lectin-free diets, Mediterranean, low-carb, low-fat, gluten-free, and more—mostly adhere to a whole foods approach and remove harmful ultra-processed foods and include protective foods.

Perhaps the real focus should be on shifting people from an obesogenic, disease-causing, nutrient-depleted diet to one rich in whole foods and protective foods that promote weight loss, health, and well-being. That, my friends, is the goal of the Pegan Diet.

Why is this more important than ever? Our modern industrial diet is currently the biggest killer on the planet, exceeding smoking and every other cause. Conservatively our modern diet, rich in processed foods made from wheat (white flour), corn (high-fructose corn syrup and many industrial food additives), and soy (soybean oil), and lacking in protective, healing whole foods (fruits, vegetables, nuts, seeds, whole grains, beans, seafood, etc.), kills 11 million people a year. I believe that is a gross underestimate. Each year about 57 million people die around the world. Three-quarters of those deaths (or 42 million) are due to chronic diseases such as heart disease, diabetes, cancer, and dementia, mostly caused by poor diet. Even infectious diseases, like COVID-19, are more likely to sicken and kill those who are overweight or suffer from chronic disease. The costs are staggering. In the United States, the direct and indirect cost for chronic disease is projected to be $95 trillion over the next 35 years, or about 1 in 5 dollars of our entire economy. Globally it's much more, and getting worse as we export our American diet to every part of the globe.

If we want to lower the total burden of chronic disease, survive another pandemic, save our planet and communities, and create a happier, less divided society, we have to overhaul the way that we grow, produce, distribute, and consume food around the world. We have to come together, stop the diet wars, and embrace the healing power of proper nutrition. That is why I wrote this book—to showcase the power of food and present an inclusive and sustainable food philosophy.

The Pegan Diet is unique in four ways. I'll cover each foundational principle next.

THE PEGAN DIET TREATS FOOD AS MEDICINE

The first foundation is this: *Food is medicine,* with both the power to heal and the power to harm. The best strategy for a long and healthy life is to eat your medicine—get your drugs at the farmacy, not the pharmacy! Food is far more than just calories or energy to fuel our bodies. It is information, instructions that regulate every function of our bodies in real time. Remarkable discoveries over the last few decades now enable us to use food not just for pleasure, joy, connection, and nourishment but also for rejuvenation, thriving, and even reversing disease. Quality and nutrient density are foundational to building a thriving human community. Some suggest we should all be *nutrivores,* prioritizing nutrient density; others propose we become *qualitarians* and focus on quality, no matter what dietary philosophy we hold. One discovery embodied in the Pegan Diet is that we are all unique, not just in terms of our preferences but also in our biology. Our genetic and biochemical uniqueness can guide us toward *personalized nutrition.* Despite our personal beliefs, some may thrive on a vegan diet; others may wither. Some become superhuman on a Paleo diet, and others not so much. The key is to explore your biology, not stay fixed in a particular ideology.

We are just beginning to understand how food influences our cells, tissues, organs, moods, thoughts, feelings, and the structure of our bodies, but what scientists have discovered over the last few decades is astonishing. Food is not only a source of energy, joy, connection, and pleasure; it can also rejuvenate us and even reverse disease. When we think of food, we think of protein, carbohydrates, fats, fiber, vitamins, and minerals. But the most important parts of food may be the tens of thousands of medicinal compounds embedded in plants and even animal foods that regulate, modulate, and influence nearly all of the 37 billion billion chemical reactions that occur in our bodies every second. I call this process *symbiotic-phytoadaptation*. It means our bodies use chemicals found in food to beneficially influence each of our biological systems.

Through evolution, we have borrowed the molecular magic embedded in foods to optimize and supercharge our biology. For example, we can't synthesize vitamin C or omega-3 fats; we have to get these from nature. And it's not just the obvious essential fatty acids, amino acids, and vitamins and minerals we get from our food; we also get important molecules called phytochemicals.

There are 25,000-plus phytochemicals in the plant kingdom identified to date, and they've only recently been deemed critical for health. Surprisingly they are also found in animals, such as in grass-fed cows, who consume a wide array of nutrient-dense plant foods. While deficiency of these phytochemicals may not result in an acute disease like scurvy or rickets or in protein malnutrition, it can lead to long-latency deficiency diseases such as heart disease, diabetes, hypertension, obesity, dementia, depression, and more.

The only way to take advantage of these disease-fighting compounds is to focus on our food quality. Deeply colorful plant foods, organic and grass-fed meats, and wild fatty fish are abundant in compounds that protect our cells and fight off invaders. If you eat industrial food, even vegetables, your diet will be depleted. Organic vegetables are more nutrient-dense. Factory-farmed cows fed a simplified diet of corn, cow poop, candy, and ground-up animal parts produce meat that leads to inflammation and disease. Wild elk or regeneratively raised cows that forage on dozens of medical plants produce meat that has the opposite effect.

Every time you take a bite of food, consider that you are programming your biology for health or disease. When you eat healthy food, you are, in fact, eating medicine.

THE PEGAN DIET IS BASED ON FUNCTIONAL MEDICINE

The greatest discovery of the last 50 years is that food is medicine with the power to prevent, treat, and even reverse most chronic disease (and quickly). This discovery is mostly ignored by traditional medicine. Is there an approach to medicine, disease treatment, and health creation that incorporates this new understanding? Yes. It is called *functional medicine*. It is what I have been practicing for nearly 30 years with remarkable, life-changing results. Functional medicine practitioners understand that what you put at the end of your fork is more powerful than anything you will ever find in a prescription bottle. It works faster, better, and cheaper, and all the side effects are good ones.

The body is a biological ecosystem, a network of dynamically interacting, interconnected systems. In conventional medicine they might say there's a problem with your heart, liver, brain, or colon, for example. Diseases within each organ are viewed as separate and disconnected from the rest of the body. In functional medicine, we don't view the body as a collection of isolated organs; instead the body is one network of systems. Treating disease means treating these systems or treating the root causes of imbalance. Functional medicine is the science of creating health, not simply treating the symptoms.

How do you treat the root cause and create health? It's simple. Take out the bad stuff. Add the good stuff. The body's natural intelligence and healing mechanisms do the rest. We start by removing the cause (or causes) and then replacing what the body needs to thrive. Almost all diseases (other than dominant inherited genetic conditions like Down syndrome) have the same few causes: toxins (both internal and external, such as pesticides, herbicides, plastics, heavy metals, and more), allergens (environmental and food), microbes (imbalances in bacteria—especially in the microbiome—as well as viruses, parasites, worms, and ticks), and poor diet and stress (physical or psychological). These triggers of disease interact with your genes and all your basic biological networks—your gut, immune system, hormones, brain chemistry, detoxification system, energy production, circulation, and even your body's structure (cells, membranes, muscles, bones). In addition to the triggers of disease, there are necessary ingredients for health—real food, nutrients, hormones, light, water, air, rest, sleep, movement, love, connection, meaning, and purpose. These are the raw materials, each needed in proper balance, different for each individual, to create a healthy human. Creating health is simply a matter of identifying and removing the triggers and replacing the necessary ingredients.

Food, it turns out, is the biggest driver of imbalances in your biological networks and the biggest lever for rapid change, the reversal of disease, and the creation of health. While most doctors have not seen the power of food, mostly because they were not trained in using food as medicine, I have seen miracles over the decades, and so have thousands of functional medicine colleagues. I don't even like to call them miracles. They result from applying the latest advances in understanding how our bodies actually work, not how we were trained in medical school. Autoimmune diseases disappear, depression vanishes, migraines evaporate, psoriasis and eczema clear up, Alzheimer's patients' memory improves, and type 2 diabetes disappears in a few weeks. These are not anomalies or spontaneous remissions but reproducible results based on applying food as medicine with the model of functional medicine.

Food is the most important tool in my medical toolbox. It works faster, works better, and is cheaper than medication. Applying food as medicine is the foundation of functional medicine. But you don't have to see a functional medicine doctor to understand how to use food as medicine. The Pegan Diet was created to help anyone, anywhere, understand the power of nutrition and take steps to move toward better health today. You ingest pounds of foreign material into your body daily. If all calories were the same, it would not matter what you ate. But they are not. Food carries information molecules, instructions, and code that programs your biology with every bite for better or worse. Industrial food drives inflammation, triggers oxidative stress, promotes imbalances in hormone and brain chemistry, overloads your detoxification system, depletes your energy, damages your microbiome, and changes your gene expression to turn on disease-causing genes. Real, whole nutrient and phytonutrient–rich food does the opposite—turns off inflammation, increases antioxidant systems, balances hormones and brain chemistry, boosts detoxification, increases energy, optimizes your microbiome, and turns on disease-preventing, health-promoting genes.

Food impacts all these core systems or networks in the body. The Pegan Diet combines the latest science of food as medicine and strategies to optimize these systems into a practical way of eating for life.

THE PEGAN DIET SAVES YOU AND THE PLANET

Eating is an agricultural, environmental, and political act, not just a personal one. What we eat affects how food is grown, which food is grown, and which agricultural methods are used. Is our food grown in ways that produce the most nutrient-dense food, conserve water, build soil, reverse climate change, and increase the biodiversity of plants, insects, and animals? Or does it produce food that drives sickness and environmental destruction? Simply put, the Pegan Diet is a *regenerative diet*—one that regenerates human and planetary health. In other words, no matter what dietary approach we choose, we should all be *regenetarians*. That is something 1 believe we can all agree on. A diet that heals us, heals the environment and reverses climate change. Becoming a regenetarian might just save you and the world.

The food system is the number one cause of climate change, depletion of soil (we have sixty harvests left, according to the UN) and fresh water, and the loss of biodiversity of plants, animals, pollinators, insects, and even the microbiology of the soil. Our food system, which involves deforestation, soil erosion, factory farming of animals, agrochemical damage to the land, transport, refrigeration, and food waste, contributes about 50 percent of all greenhouse gas emissions. For example, soil is the biggest carbon sink on the planet, far greater than rainforests. It can hold 3 times the amount of carbon currently in the atmosphere, which is 1 trillion tons. In fact, of that 1 trillion tons of carbon driving climate change, one-third comes from the loss of soil carbon through erosion and destruction of soil life. The 400 billion pounds of nitrogen fertilizers are another major driver of climate change. They require about 2 percent of all global fossil fuel production to produce (mostly as fracking-derived natural gas). When applied to the soil, nitrogen fertilizers kill the microbial life and produce nitrous oxide, a greenhouse gas 300 times more potent than carbon dioxide.

These problems start with our food system, and so do the solutions. I have detailed both the problems and the solutions in my book *Food Fix: How to Save Our Health, Our Communities, and Our Planet— One Bite at a Time.* And I am working to change the policies that drive the system with the Food Fix Campaign (foodfix.org). The critical first step is to become a regenetarian (more on that in Principle 9: Eat Like a Regenetarian). The more people demand change, the more the system will change.

Large companies have stepped in where the government has not, funding conventional farmers to convert their farms to regenerative agriculture. This way of producing food is the antidote to our current farming system, which produces massive quantities of commodity crops that sicken humans and the planet. Regenerative agriculture raises food in a way that restores soil, conserves water, increases biodiversity, reverses climate change, produces more nutrient-dense, phytonutrient-rich quality food, all while making farmers far more money and making their farms resistant to drought, floods, and climate impacts. In short, it stops the cycle of destruction.

The large agribusiness companies frighten us by making us believe that we cannot feed the growing global population without them. The science does not support this claim. In fact, localized regenerative farming ecosystems are scalable globally and are the only true solution to food production in the future. Regenerative agriculture is the future of food. And each of us can play a role.

THE PEGAN DIET IS AN INCLUSIVE, FLEXIBLE WAY OF EATING FOR LIFE

Finally, the Pegan Diet is a way to eat for life. Most diets fail because they are restrictive, confusing, and leave us feeling ashamed when we fall off the wagon. The Pegan Diet is sustainable because it's not about being perfect; it's about feeding your body nutritionally dense food 90 percent of the time and leaving room for pleasure foods and treats (but still real-food treats). I am not perfect, and I don't expect anyone else to be either. We all have families, social events, parties where we want to enjoy a margarita and a slice of cake. We can feed ourselves well, take care of our bodies, *and* enjoy life's pleasures. Setting yourself up for success involves incorporating the right habits, getting the family involved, and learning to cook, which I promise can become anyone's favorite activity.

I've tried nearly every diet on myself (and my patients). I've been vegan, Paleo, high-fat, low-fat, raw food, you name it. What I've come to learn is that you don't have to define your diet. Instead, do what makes you feel good. Listen to *your* body. In the Pegan Diet I have created a set of simple, sane principles to guide you, but I hope that we will all eat this way one day without needing to give it a name. I want the Pegan Diet to be sustainable for anyone, anywhere. If you eat meat, you can follow this diet. If you don't eat meat, you can follow these principles. If you're just getting started on your health journey, it's a great place to begin! If you've experimented with many diets but are still frustrated or confused or don't feel well, this is for you.

Eating is the most important act we perform every day. It's an act that connects us to nature, ecological cycles, biological functions, and, of course, one another. We are part of a great web of nature that provides the raw materials for creating a vibrant, healthy life.

In the following pages, you'll find 21 Practical Principles for Reclaiming Your Health in a Nutritionally Confusing

World. These principles provide a road map, guiding you toward a personalized approach to eating in a way that is good for you, your family, your community, and the planet. And, more importantly, that is delicious, nourishing, and joyful.

PRINCIPLE 1

Use Food as Your Farmacy

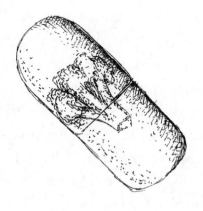

Plant and animal foods have a wide array of molecules that influence every aspect of our biology: proteins; fats; carbohydrates; vitamins; minerals; soluble, insoluble, and resistant fibers; prebiotics; probiotics; antioxidants; phytochemicals; and even microRNA, the genetic material of plants, which we absorb and which communicates with our own DNA. Foods are made not of ingredients but of complex compounds, all dynamically influencing your biology. Think about the implications of every single bite of food you eat. You are literally programming your biological software for better or worse. Most don't understand the link between what they eat and how they feel, or between food and the myriad ailments to which humans are prone. This lack of understanding has resulted in a growing dependence on doctors, prescriptions, and ultimately hospitals to rescue them from damaging food choices. If you learn to view food as instructions that influence every aspect of your biology, and learn to combine that knowledge with the joy of cooking, there will be only pleasure and healing.

Functional medicine, the science of creating health, focuses on the root cause of disease, and food almost always plays a role in both the cause and the cure. If a doctor sees a patient complaining of hopelessness, sadness, trouble sleeping, low sex drive, and lack of appetite, the doctor will diagnose depression. But "depression" is just the name we give to people who share those symptoms. It says nothing about the causes of the symptoms, which could be many. The treatment prescribed is an antidepressant, but depression is not a Prozac deficiency. In conventional medicine, thinking stops at the diagnosis. In functional medicine, thinking starts at the diagnosis. Depression, for example, may be caused by low thyroid function, celiac disease, B_{12} deficiency, vitamin D deficiency, antibiotics that alter the microbiome, heavy metal toxicity, omega-3 deficiency, or even insulin resistance (from too much starch and sugar). Each of these causes requires a very different treatment.

In functional medicine, we don't divide the body into separate organs; we look at the functioning of seven different systems. Nearly every one of the 155,000 diseases listed in the disease classification system known as ICD-10 is caused by imbalances in these seven interconnected systems. Fix those systems and you fix the problem. How do you do that? You start with food. You can eat to reverse deficiencies. You can eat to heal your gut, reduce inflammation, enhance your immune function, balance your hormones, and boost your detoxification system. You can eat to strengthen your bones and your muscles.

In Principle 1, I'm going to give you an overview of each of the seven systems in functional medicine and how you can use food as medicine, or as I like to say, your farmacy.

THE GUT MICROBIOME

Your gut microbiome, the magical kingdom of microbes living in you, may be the most important organ in your body. An unhealthy microbiome can cause heart disease, cancer, diabetes, obesity, autism, autoimmunity, dementia, allergies, asthma, fibromyalgia, Parkinson's, and skin disorders like acne, eczema, and psoriasis, not to mention all the digestive disorders, including irritable bowel, reflux, and colitis.[1] Bad bugs in our gut grow for two reasons: not eating enough of the foods that feed the good guys, and eating too many gut-busting foods. The biggest culprit when it comes to harming the gut is gluten. Modern wheat has an excess of powerful inflammatory proteins called gliadins that create a leaky gut, driving inflammation and imbalances in the gut flora. Leaky gut is also called increased intestinal permeability. The surface area of your intestinal lining is the size of a tennis court. And it is only one cell thick—one cell between you and a sewer! The glue that holds all the intestinal cells breaks down, creating little holes that allow food proteins and bacterial products to "leak" into the bloodstream and interact with the immune system (60 percent of which is right below the intestinal lining). This causes inflammation in every system of the body. Sugar, excessive starch, processed foods, and refined vegetable oils also feed the bad bugs and lead to leaky gut and inflammation throughout the body, causing many chronic diseases. Sugar, starch, and bad fats. These are what America and most of the world eats. They're about 60 percent of our calories.

Is there a gut-healing diet? Absolutely. First, good bugs need all types of fiber to thrive. The most essential fibers are called prebiotics. Certain foods have high levels, including artichokes, asparagus, plantains, seaweed, and more. All fiber-rich foods will help keep your inner garden healthy — vegetables, fruits, nuts, seeds, whole grains, and beans.

In addition to fiber, probiotics are critical for healthy gut function. You might take a probiotic supplement, but you can get probiotics from fermented foods like sauerkraut, pickles, tempeh, miso, natto, and kimchi.

Your gut also needs specific nutrients to function well. Zinc, in foods like pumpkin seeds and oysters, is necessary for digestive enzyme function. Omega-3 fats from fish, such as sardines and herring, are needed to regulate inflammation and heal leaky gut. Vitamin A, from sources like beef liver, cod liver, salmon, and goat cheese, is also necessary for gut healing and regulating gut immune function. Foods with collagen, such as bone broth, contain *glycosaminoglycans,* which help heal the gut. Kudzu, a Japanese root, is a powerful gut-soothing food.

In Principle 15, I'll share new research about the role of polyphenols in gut health and how to start a gut-healing protocol. Food is the most important regulator of your microbiome. If you feed your gut well, you'll set yourself up for optimal health.

THE IMMUNE SYSTEM AND INFLAMMATORY SYSTEM

Immunity has been top of mind for all of us since we started to see the frightening effects of COVID-19 in 2020. Those who are obese or chronically ill (both states of inflammation) are most at risk for severe illness and death. What foods make them pre-inflamed and cause chronic disease? The same foods damage each system in the body—bad fats, refined sugars, excessive starches, processed foods, conventional dairy, and poor-quality food all drive inflammation. Sugar and starch are hidden in all processed food. They create a chain reaction, causing blood sugar to spike, which causes insulin to spike, leading to insulin resistance. The more sugar and starch you eat, the higher your insulin levels. More insulin, more fat storage, more inflammation, more hunger, more immune suppression. The loss of healthy gut flora, an excess of gut-busting foods, and reliance on medications collectively result in leaky gut, which causes a rise in food sensitivities and food allergies—all of which drive inflammation. The most common food sensitivities are gluten and dairy.

The solution: Cut down on starch and sugar, try an elimination diet (three weeks off gluten and dairy), and focus on anti-inflammatory foods. Many of the 25,000-plus phytochemicals in food are potent anti-inflammatories. Where is the best place to find these compounds? Fruits and vegetables. Foods like spices and certain oils also contain powerful anti-inflammatories. Extra virgin olive oil contains oleocanthal, for example, which activates the same anti-inflammatory receptors as ibuprofen without all the side effects. Using turmeric, ginger, and rosemary with your meat can neutralize potential inflammation.[2] Omega-3 fatty acids found in wild foods like fish, seafood, and some nuts and seeds are essential for proper immune function. Mushrooms, including shiitake, maitake, reishi, chaga, turkey tail, and cordyceps, contain immune-regulating and anti-cancer compounds called polysaccharides. And foods rich in vitamins and minerals boost immunity and reduce inflammation, including vitamin C, zinc, selenium, and vitamin D. Vitamin D alone regulates hundreds of genes that affect inflammation and immunity. So a meal of guavas and parsley (vitamin C), pumpkin seeds and oysters (zinc), Brazil nuts and sardines (selenium), and porcini mushrooms and herring (vitamin D) is an immune-boosting, anti-inflammatory super meal! I don't know what anyone would make with all of these ingredients, but you get the idea. Try to include more of these immune-supporting foods daily.

THE ENERGY SYSTEM

The energy stored in food in the form of fats, protein, and carbohydrates gets combined with oxygen in the tiny little factories inside your cells called *mitochondria*. The food and oxygen then produce the form of energy used by our bodies called ATP. It powers everything. Once we stop producing energy, we die. Some foods burn clean, while others create a lot of exhaust that damages our tissues and cells and produces free radicals that cause oxidation (similar to rusting) and inflammation. Our bodies produce their own antioxidants to protect us from this damage. When we overeat processed foods, our antioxidant systems can't keep up.

To make energy from food and oxygen, the assembly line in your mitochondria needs specific vitamins, minerals, and other nutrients: B vitamins, coenzyme Q10, carnitine, zinc, magnesium, selenium, omega-3 fats, lipoic acid, N-acetylcysteine, vitamin E, vitamin K, sulfur, and others. Our modern nutrient-depleted diet provides very few of these mitochondrial boosters. How do we shift from an energy-lacking diet to an energy-producing one? Eat foods like blueberries, pomegranate seeds, grass-fed beef and butter, broccoli, sardines, extra virgin olive oil, avocados, and almonds. One of the best fuel sources for the mitochondria is MCT oil (medium-chain triglycerides), found in unrefined coconut oil. It is the cleanest-burning preferred fuel for your mitochondria and an excellent performance enhancer before exercise. I sometimes add a tablespoon of MCT oil to my morning coffee to sustain energy and enhance brain function.

THE DETOXIFICATION SYSTEM

When we hear "detox," most of us think of drug or alcohol rehab or fad "cleansing" diets. But the body has a very sophisticated detoxification system to handle internal waste and environmental toxins. Imagine if your toilet backed up for a week or if your sink were clogged up for a few days. The same things happen in your body when your detoxification system fails. If your liver fails, you can't process waste and need a liver transplant. If your kidneys stop working, you get very sick and die in a week or two without dialysis. If your colon is clogged up, well, you get the idea! Sadly, in this modern world, we are exposed to more toxins than ever before from harmful chemicals in food, water, air, household products, cosmetics, and more. Thankfully our biology is designed to process waste and toxins. We just have to take extra care to support our detoxification system on a day-to-day basis.

The first step to enhancing detoxification is to drink clean, filtered water. Water helps remove waste through the kidneys and gut. Fiber is essential for helping waste products get through our colon quickly. Our liver, however, needs extra help. The liver has many pathways to removing toxins from the body with fancy names like methylation, glucuronidation, acetylation, and glutathione conjugation, and each of these pathways needs support. The food group that best boosts our detox pathways is the cruciferous vegetable family (broccoli, collards, kale, cabbage, Brussels sprouts). This family contains compounds with sulfur that enhance the production of glutathione, the body's master antioxidant. Garlic and onions also provide the sulfur needed for detoxification. Adequate amino acids from protein are essential to fuel these pathways. Green tea is a super detoxifier, which may be why the Japanese can handle the mercury overload from too much sushi. Green tea chelates (binds) heavy metals. The liver needs adequate levels of B_1, B_2, B_3, B_6, B_{12}, folate, manganese, magnesium, zinc, and selenium to facilitate all the chemical reactions needed for detoxification. These nutrients are found in animal protein, seafood, nuts, seeds, and green vegetables. The liver also needs a rich array of phytochemicals, including flavonoids, and compounds found in herbs and spices. Curcumin, found in the Indian spice turmeric, is a superfood that reduces inflammation and oxidative stress and aids detoxification.[3] Rosemary, ginger, cilantro, dandelion greens, parsley, lemon peel, watercress, burdock root, and artichokes are all powerful detoxifying foods to add to your diet regularly.

THE CIRCULATORY SYSTEM

The biggest killer in the world today is cardiovascular disease, mostly caused by insulin resistance, prediabetes, or type 2 diabetes. Clogged arteries can lead to heart attacks, strokes, amputations in diabetics, and even dementia. Contrary to popular understanding, this is not a plumbing problem that can be fixed by bypass or Roto-Rooter treatments such as angioplasty or stents. Cholesterol alone isn't the problem. The problem occurs when our body is inflamed, turning cholesterol into fragile plaques that coat our arteries. Unfortunately, the Standard American Diet is riddled with inflammatory foods like bad fats, bad meat, sugar, and starches. For example, studies show that a single fast-food meal harms blood vessels.[4] The good news is that phytonutrients[5] and antioxidants[6] have been shown to help reduce the effects of ultra-processed food. This doesn't mean you can eat fast food as long as you also eat the good stuff. It means focus on foods rich in phytonutrients and antioxidants and eat less (or none) of the disease-causing foods.

The other important foods for vascular health are foods

that increase nitric oxide, or NO, a molecule that helps increase blood flow. The amino acid arginine is the precursor for NO, and the best food sources are pumpkin seeds, sesame seeds, walnuts, almonds, turkey breast, soybeans, and seaweed. Omega-3 fats from wild fish also help improve blood vessel health, and they prevent clotting.[7] We've all been told that olive oil is one of the most heart-healthy foods on the planet. It turns out that the benefits of olive oil are likely due to the effect of polyphenols on endothelial function and on reducing blood vessel inflammation.[8] These are just a few examples of how food can protect against one of the deadliest diseases in the world.

THE COMMUNICATION SYSTEM: HORMONES AND NEUROTRANSMITTERS

We have a beautifully tuned communication system constantly sending messages around the body. This communication system includes our hormones and neurotransmitters. When they play out of tune, like instruments in a symphony orchestra, disease happens. Depression, anxiety, insulin resistance, chronic fatigue. Premenstrual syndrome, polycystic ovarian syndrome, sexual dysfunction. Breast, cervical, and uterine cancer. Low libido and erectile dysfunction. You get the picture. It's not pretty.

I have written many books about hormones and food. The single biggest hormonal disorder we face is insulin resistance. One in two Americans has prediabetes or type 2 diabetes, and 75 percent are overweight. This is the result of the mountains of sugar and flour we consume, which leads to high glucose and insulin, which creates a domino effect. It drives excess calories into fat cells that then produce messengers to increase hunger, slow metabolism, prevent fat burning, and cause inflammation to spike. In women, too much insulin turns estrogen into testosterone. This can lead to something misleadingly called polycystic ovarian syndrome. It is not an ovarian problem. It is a dietary problem. The extra testosterone in women causes hair loss, facial hair, acne, and infertility. In men, the testosterone gets converted to estrogen, which is why men with big bellies often have man boobs and lose the hair on their bodies. The same high-sugar and -starch diet also spikes the hormones cortisol and adrenaline. When you eat a sugar- and starch-laden diet, your body literally perceives it as a stressor, just like when a tiger chases you. Adrenaline and cortisol increase, worsening insulin resistance and increasing cravings for sugar and starch.

In my practice I bring balance to hormones by addressing insulin resistance, first using the Pegan Diet—a whole foods, good-fat, plant-rich, fiber-rich, low-glycemic diet. For women who are dealing with estrogen dominance (leading to PMS and cancers), I work on maintaining a healthy gut microbiome by increasing fibers (such as flaxseeds), which can detoxify and remove excess estrogen. For men who have low testosterone, we reduce sugar and increase healthy fats. I raised my testosterone significantly when I reduced starches and ate more healthy fats from nuts, seeds, avocado, olive oil, and grass-fed meats.

Thyroid function is also affected by what we eat. Our thyroid regulates most functions in the body related to metabolism, energy, and even hormones. One in ten men and one in five women have low thyroid function. Low thyroid function can be triggered by gluten, too many raw kale smoothies (raw cruciferous veggies can block thyroid function), and diets low in zinc, selenium, vitamin D, and iodine. Environmental toxins often found in our food, such as pesticides and mercury, also damage our thyroid. Adding foods rich in zinc (pumpkin seeds and oysters), selenium (sardines and Brazil nuts), vitamin D (herring and porcini mushrooms), and iodine (seaweed and fish) can help optimize thyroid function.

These are just a few examples of the ways in which food impacts our hormones. The Pegan Diet is essential to good communication and balance among all our cells and systems.

THE CELL MEMBRANE AND MUSCULOSKELETAL STRUCTURE

Every cell in our body turns over every seven years. Some turn over daily, some weekly, and some take longer. Ever wonder how we make new cells, organs, tissues, skin, muscles, bone, and even brain cells? We don't just manufacture them from thin air. The raw materials all come from what we eat. Do you want to be made of Doritos or grass-fed steak? Coca-Cola or wild blueberries? Our body's structure, which determines our functioning, is dependent on food to provide the building blocks—the proteins, fats, and minerals that make up who we are. Funnily enough, we are not made of carbohydrates, and they are not considered an essential nutrient. If you are a healthy, lean female, your body is made up of 55 percent water, 16 percent protein, 23 percent fat, 6 percent minerals, less than 1 percent carbohydrate, and small amounts of vitamins. The problem is that our processed diet is about 50 to 60 percent carbohydrate, mostly low-quality refined starches and sugars that are the raw materials for processed food.

To support our cells, organs, muscles, and bones, we need the best-quality foods. We need to eat healthy fats—our brain is 60 percent fat, our nerve coverings are all made from fat, every one of our 10 trillion cells is wrapped in a little fatty membrane. We need quality protein. The body makes most of its important molecules from protein—including muscle, cells, and immune molecules. The best type of protein to build muscle is other muscle: animal protein. You can get protein from plant foods, but the quality is lower, and plants have lower levels of key amino acids (branched-chain amino acids such as leucine) needed to synthesize new muscle. We'll talk about this more in Principle 14. Finally, we need all of the vitamins and minerals required to build tissues, muscles, and bones, including vitamin D, vitamin K, calcium, magnesium, and more.

PRINCIPLE 1 TAKEAWAY

Every level of your health is impacted by what you eat. You can eat to build muscle, build healthy bones, gain energy, balance your hormones, fix your gut, boost your immunity, improve heart health, and everything in between. Next time you chomp down on something, ask yourself if you are fine with it becoming part of you for the long term. If not, don't eat it and seek out the best-quality ingredients instead (and by the way, taste and quality go together). Everything (our health, our communities, our planet) is connected to what we eat (or don't). As we move through the rest of the principles of the Pegan Diet, infused with the science of functional medicine, you'll learn practical ways to use food as your farmacy.

Eat the Rainbow

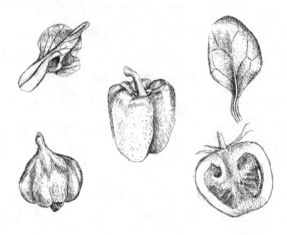

My friend Michael Pollan says, "Eat food, not too much, mostly plants." The foundation of any healthy way of eating, including the Pegan Diet, is to make it plant-rich. Notice I said plant-rich, not plant-based. Plant-rich means that the bulk of your diet consists of plant foods with the addition of adequate high-quality protein and healthy fats. Plant foods are nutrient-dense—lots of nutrients, few calories. They contain two unique ingredients: fiber and phytonutrients. It turns out these two components found uniquely in plants are critically necessary to optimize your gut microbiome and to create healthy functioning in every system of your body. You won't get a deficiency disease like scurvy or rickets without them, but you will likely get a chronic disease.

THE POWER OF PHYTOCHEMICALS

If food is medicine, think of plant foods as the most powerful medicine in your farmacy, with the vast array of colors representing more than 25,000 beneficial chemicals. You may have heard of these phytochemicals or phytonutrients before. They include polyphenols, resveratrol, flavonoids, isoflavonoids, terpenoids, and carotenoids, to name a few, and they play a significant role in creating optimal health and disease prevention. These compounds benefit our biology in hundreds of ways. They boost immunity, reduce inflammation, and have anti-cancer and anti-aging effects.[9] Take broccoli, for example, worthy of its health-promoting reputation. It's a phytochemical powerhouse full of sulforaphane, glucosinolates, chlorophyll, carotenoids — all disease- and cancer-fighting, antioxidant, detoxifying compounds.[10] Studies have shown that eating 2 cups of broccoli a week can reduce cancer risk. The compounds in broccoli can also help lower bad cholesterol, improve digestion and eye health, and reduce overall inflammation in the body. What may surprise you is that these phytochemicals are found in animal foods in significant amounts when the animals are free to forage on a multitude of grasses and wild plants (see Principle 5).

Why are plants so rich in phytochemicals? They don't make them for our benefit, even though we hijack them to optimize our biology. The phytochemicals found in the edible plant kingdom are the plants' messaging system, a means of protection, defense, and survival. These compounds deter pests, prevent the plants from being eaten, increase hardiness, and even communicate messages to other plants, animals, and the trillions of microbes and fungi found within the soil. Antioxidant, anti-inflammatory, detoxifying, anti-cancer, and disease-fighting medicines proclaim themselves through their bright colors. We should all eat the rainbow of colors (except Skittles and M&Ms) regularly—red, green, yellow, orange, and purple plants, even the weird ones we've never tried before.

Think of all of the colorful plant foods that you see in the supermarket and the hundreds of plants that we could eat. Our hunter-gatherer ancestors ate more than 800 varieties of plant foods. Today, fifteen crops make up 90 percent of our food intake, and globally three crops make up two-thirds of our calories—wheat, corn, and rice.

The US dietary guidelines recommend a minimum of 3 cups of veggies per day (or 5 to 9 servings of fruits and vegetables, where a serving is half a cup). The optimal amount should be 6 to 8 cups or 12 to 18 servings. Only 0.9 percent of teenagers, 2.2 percent of men, and 3.5 percent of women consume the recommended amounts. The veggies Americans love do not qualify as medicinal powerhouses—not even close. The top five vegetables are potatoes (as French fries), tomatoes (as ketchup), onions, iceberg lettuce, and corn. Except for onions, not the healthiest bunch!

We understand that fruits and vegetables are good for us, but many of us don't understand which ones to eat or why. Principle 2 is a crash course in understanding how medicinal compounds that aid in healing are expressed through the colors of the rainbow.

COLORS OF FRUITS AND VEGETABLES AND THEIR PROPERTIES[11]

Color	Foods	Phytochemicals	Benefits
Red	Apples, tomatoes, blood oranges, cherries, cranberries, pink grapefruit, pomegranate, raspberries, red currants, red pears, red plums, strawberries, watermelon, radicchio, radishes, red beets, red bell peppers, red cabbage, red chard, red onion	Anthocyanins, carotenoids, ellagic acid, ellagitannins, flavones, lycopene, phloretin, quercetin	Anti-inflammatory, general antioxidant activity, immune modulation
Orange	Apricots, oranges, cantaloupe, kumquat, mandarins, mangoes, nectarines, oranges, papaya, passion fruit, peaches, persimmons, tangerines, carrots, orange bell peppers, pumpkin, sweet potatoes, turmeric, yams	Alpha-carotene, beta-carotene, beta-cryptoxanthin, bioflavonoids, carotenoids, curcuminoids	Antioxidants for fat-soluble tissues, endocrine modulation, fertility support
Yellow	Asian pears, lemons, pineapple, banana, star fruit, potatoes, squash (acorn, buttercup, butternut, summer, winter), yellow bell peppers, yellow onions	Gingerol, lutein, nobiletin, prebiotic fibers, rutin, zeaxanthin	Gastric motility and regulation, glycemic impact, supporting gut microbiome
Green	Avocado, Brussels sprouts, green apples, limes, olives, pears, artichokes, asparagus, bell peppers, bok choy, broccoli, cabbage, celery, cucumbers, edamame, green beans, greens (beet, chard, collards, dandelion, kale, lettuce, mustard, spinach, turnip), okra, rosemary and other herbs, snow peas, watercress	Oleuropein, phytosterols, silymarin, sulforaphane, tannins, theaflavins, tyrosol, vitexin	Antioxidant, blood vessel support, supports healthy circulation and methylation
Blue	Blackberries, blueberries, boysenberries, figs, huckleberries, prunes, purple grapes, raisins, eggplant, plums, purple bell peppers, purple carrots, purple cauliflower, purple kale, purple potatoes	Anthocyanidins, flavonoids, phenolic acids, proanthocyanidins, pterostilbene, resveratrol, stilbenes	Antioxidant, cognitive support, healthy mood balance, role in neuronal health

There are at least seventy different foods listed on this chart. When it comes to eating our medicine, the options are endless. Yet many of us stick to the same three or four fruits and vegetables every week—bananas, oranges, iceberg or romaine lettuce. I encourage you to expand your diet of fruits and veggies to include colorful nutritional powerhouses.

If you're struggling with diabetes, belly fat, weight loss challenges, or gut dysbiosis, you might need to focus on low-glycemic fruits and vegetables. Seek out ones that are low in sugar and high in phytonutrients, like berries, and limit your fruit to half a cup a day or one piece of fruit per day. The perfect scale for food would combine nutrient density with glycemic load. Fruits like grapes, bananas, and dried fruit rank high on the glycemic load scale. If you're not struggling with gut dysfunction, belly fat, or diabetes, enjoy these fruits from time to time, but not as staples. Instead, focus on fruits like berries, apples, kiwi, and pomegranate, about half a cup once or twice a day.

Some of the best fruits have very little sugar and include beneficial fats: coconuts, avocados, and olives. I call these fat fruits. Avocados and olives are heart-healthy, and coconuts contain medium-chain triglycerides, which can boost brain function and metabolism. These are some of my favorite overlooked fruits and fats.

When it comes to veggies, go crazy. I often make three veggie dishes with every meal—an artichoke, a salad, and sautéed broccolini, for example. We'll dive into vegetables a little more in the next principle since they are the most essential part of your diet. For now, know that almost every meal is made more nutritious by adding more vegetables.

DOES ORGANIC MATTER?

Buying organic fruits and vegetables is important for your health, but it can get costly. It turns out that we don't always have to buy organic. Some foods are more likely to contain pesticides than others. EWG (Environmental Working Group, ewg.org) puts out a Dirty Dozen and Clean Fifteen list every year. Follow it to know which veggies and fruits should be organic and which are okay conventionally grown. I've added the list here for your convenience.

Best to buy organic	*Okay to buy conventionally grown*
Strawberries, spinach, kale, nectarines, apples, grapes, peaches, cherries, pears, tomatoes, celery, potatoes, hot peppers	Avocados, sweet corn, pineapple, onions, papaya, sweet peas (frozen), eggplant, asparagus, cauliflower, cantaloupe, broccoli, mushrooms, cabbage, honeydew, kiwi

PRINCIPLE 2 TAKEAWAY

Try to include one color from each color category most days of the week. For example, have blue and red berries in your smoothie, leafy greens with your lunch, purple carrots and orange and yellow bell peppers at dinner. Eating the rainbow is your gateway to using food as medicine.

Follow the 75 Percent Rule

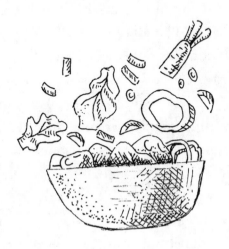

Did you know that all plant foods are carbohydrates? They're whole plant food carbohydrates, or what I like to call "slow carbs." The difference between whole plant food carbohydrates and refined carbohydrates is that refined carbs are stripped of their nutritive value and send your blood sugar on a roller coaster, whereas plant food carbs are rich in vitamins, minerals, fiber, and phytochemicals and help balance your blood sugar, providing medicinal compounds that optimize every single aspect of your biology. Unfortunately, our modern diet is rich in damaging refined carbs—pizza, fries, bread, pasta. These are the types of nutrient-stripped foods that drive high blood sugar, inflammation, and insulin; raise your triglycerides; lower your good cholesterol; and fuel diabetes, cancer, dementia, and heart disease. So when I tell my patients, don't fear carbs, I mean slow carbs, especially veggies—for instance, arugula, kale, broccoli, bok choy, artichokes, cucumbers, peppers, and asparagus.

Another way to think about this is to consider the glycemic load of carbs. The glycemic load indicates how a food will impact blood sugar. Processed carbohydrates rank high on the glycemic load scale. Non-starchy veggies (bok choy, kale, spinach) barely register on the glycemic load scale. You want to fill 75 percent of your plate with non-starchy vegetables. In the Pegan Diet, these superfoods make up the bulk of what you eat. They contain all of the phytonutrients we discussed in Principle 2, and they are fiber-rich and won't cause your blood sugar to spike.

While still nutritious, starchy vegetables rank slightly higher on the scale and can become problematic when overconsumed. For my patients who are diabetic, prediabetic, or struggling with weight gain, I recommend limiting starchy vegetables to half a cup up to three times a week.

Here's an easy cheat sheet to help you understand which veggies should take center stage, and which should take a back seat.

Non-starchy veggies (eat unlimited amounts)

Broccoli	Bok choy
Salad greens (arugula, kale, spinach, endive, radicchio, chard)	Brussels sprouts
	Peppers
	Tomatoes

Asparagus

Cauliflower

Okra

Mushrooms

Celery

Cucumbers

Radishes

Zucchini

Beet greens

Carrots

Sea vegetables like
seaweed

Garlic, shallots, onion

Jerusalem artichokes

Those are just a few. There are so many more!

Starchy veggies (up to ½ cup per day or less)

Sweet potatoes

Yams

Butternut squash or any
winter squashes

Pumpkin

Potatoes (fingerling
potatoes and purple
potatoes have more
phytonutrients and a
lower glycemic load
than regular white
potatoes)

If the bulk of your diet comes from non-starchy veggies, you are setting yourself up for success. Cooking new plants and incorporating them into your diet can be intimidating for many, but in this digital age, we have many resources at our fingertips. If I want to try cooking with a new ingredient, I go straight to Google and find a recipe that appeals to me. It works nine times out of ten. My mom always said, "If you do not like veggies, you probably don't know how to prepare them properly." Use the recipes in this book or go online. Eventually you'll be confident enough to try recipe-free cooking.

CAN A HIGH-FIBER DIET EXACERBATE GUT IMBALANCES?

I often talk to patients who tell me that eating too many veggies causes symptoms like bloating, gas, and diarrhea. If your stomach prevents you from eating a healthy diet, it's time to fix your stomach. Short-term dietary restrictions to heal the gut are often needed. The most common reason for gut issues is SIBO (small intestinal bacterial overgrowth), which leads to bloating and gas after eating, or what I like to call a "food baby." Through limiting certain foods for a while, like grains, beans, starchy veggies, and raw food, and doing a gut reset that clears out bad bugs and adds good ones, the gut can heal, and your diet can expand. If this is you, it's best to work with a functional medicine practitioner, dietician, or nutritionist to help create a nutrient-dense plan while you're healing. It's 100 percent possible to be Pegan while eating a lower-fiber diet, but ultimately the goal is to improve your gut so you can tolerate more fiber. Remember, the Pegan Diet is all about real food. You can still choose real, whole food even if you can't eat a ton of vegetables right now. Think clean protein like grass-fed beef or lamb, wild fatty fish, organic poultry, and cooked veggies. Also, eat plenty of healthy fats from avocado, extra virgin olive oil, and nuts and seeds if you can tolerate them. Talk to your practitioner about slowly incorporating fiber-rich foods.

PRINCIPLE 3 TAKEAWAYS

1. **Fill 75 percent of your plate with non-starchy veggies.**
   People get nervous when they hear me say this, but it's important to note that when I say that vegetables should take up 75 percent of your plate, I mean by volume, not calories.

Even if you loaded up two plates with non-starchy veggies, that would not make up the bulk of your calories if you're eating them with fats and protein. A few handfuls of greens can easily cover a plate.

2. **Eat more than the recommended serving.** While the minimum recommended amount of veggies is 5 to 9 servings (½ cup per serving), I recommend 6 to 8 cups of vegetables (or 12 to 18 servings). You can even blend them in soups or veggie smoothies. Try to include as much variety as possible. Add ½ cup of starchy vegetables a day if you'd like. If you are prediabetic or diabetic, limit starchy vegetables to ½ cup up to three times a week depending on your blood sugar.

Eat the Right Beans, Whole Grains, Nuts, and Seeds

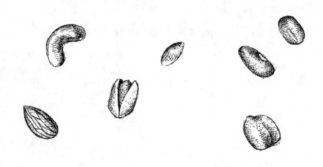

For foods that most agree are healthy, beans, grains, nuts, and seeds stir up a lot of debate between Paleo enthusiasts and vegans. For the most part, nutrition experts agree that these foods get a universal thumbs-up. However, some camps argue that lectins and phytic acid, two potentially gut-damaging compounds in beans, grains, nuts, and seeds, are not worth the benefits. Others believe that the omega-6 fats in nuts and seeds drive up inflammation and that these foods are too fatty. Some argue that beans (or legumes) contain too many carbohydrates and not enough protein. (You have to eat 2 cups of cooked pinto beans to get 24 grams of protein, but that comes with 70 grams of carbs; 4 ounces of salmon has all the protein and none of the carbs.) And as for grains, well, grain-based products have become the most popular food items since the 1992 Food Pyramid told us to eat 6 to 11 servings a day! So began our obsession with bread, pasta, rice, and cereal. Along with this obsession came a dramatic spike in insulin resistance, metabolic syndrome, type 2 diabetes, and obesity. In 1960 only 5 percent of us were obese; now over 40 percent are, an eightfold increase!

Where does the Pegan Diet stand on each? It all comes down to quality and preparation.

NUTS AND SEEDS

Nuts actually help you lose weight, but as with anything else, the dose matters. I'm not talking about a nutapalooza here. Two to four handfuls a day is great for your waistline and long-term health, including prevention of heart disease and diabetes.[12] If you're worried about nuts being fattening, know this: Not all calories are created equal. Two hundred calories from nuts and seeds is entirely different from 200 calories from a box of cookies. As for lectins, if you have a leaky gut, digestive issues, or systemic inflammation, you may benefit from a low-lectin diet. Healing your gut with a functional medicine practitioner can prevent adverse food reactions and expand your food choices.

Phytic acid, found in some nuts and seeds, can limit the absorption of vitamins and minerals. The trick is to soak raw nuts and seeds overnight and lightly toast them, which reduces the amount of lectins and phytic acid and increases your body's ability to process these foods.

Finally, there's the issue of omega-6 fats. We need these essential fats, but not from the gallons of refined oils we consume every year in processed and fried foods. Wild foods are high in omega-3 and lower in omega-6 fats. As hunter-gatherers, we consumed a ratio between 1 to 1 and 3 to 1 of omega-6 to omega-3 fats. Now, on a junk food, fast-food diet, that ratio can get as high as 20 to 1. Not only do nuts and seeds contain a nice balance of omega-3 and omega-6 fats, but they're also loaded with vitamins, fiber, protein, carbohydrates, minerals, and antioxidants like vitamin E, which prevent oxidation of the fats. Walnuts, flaxseeds, hemp seeds, and chia seeds are some of the richest sources of plant-based omega-3 fats.

A trial of a nut- and seed-free diet may be useful for certain medical conditions, such as autoimmune disease. But for most of us, nuts and seeds are nutritional and disease-fighting powerhouse superfoods.

ARE NUT FLOURS HEALTHY?

Flours made with almonds, hazelnuts, coconut, and hemp seeds are better than whole grain flours. With that being said, when you turn anything into flour, it is no longer considered a whole food. When nuts and seeds are milled, our bodies respond differently compared to when they are consumed in their whole food form. Almond flour won't cause your blood sugar to spike the way that regular bread does, but it's still flour. And if you use these flours in baking, you are likely to be adding some type of sugar. Have an occasional treat, but these should not be considered staples.

BEANS

Beans have some flaws, but they also have a lot of strengths. In the plus column, beans contain resistant starch, a special fiber that helps your microbiome produce beneficial fuel and anti-cancer compounds called short-chain fatty acids, such as butyrate. Butyrate has been shown to reduce cancer risk and speed up metabolism. The downside of beans is that they are carb-heavy without a huge protein payout. The best way to reap the benefits of beans is to choose the right ones.

My friend Dr. Carrie Diulus is a vegan, keto type 1 diabetic. Not easy but doable. She is thriving. She eats beans, but not any old beans: She eats lupini beans, a superfood. These are high in protein and fiber and have zero net carbs. The starch is indigestible, which means it doesn't get absorbed or make your blood sugar spike. You can buy them precooked in snack bags. Other low-starch beans and legumes include lentils, organic green peas or snow peas, black-eyed peas, and mung beans. The beans that I recommend avoiding or limiting on account of their starch content include lima beans, kidney beans, baked beans, and pinto beans.

When it comes to beans, preparation is everything. Beans can be a straight-up gut bomb (as many Paleo proponents point out) if you have gut dysbiosis or an unhealthy microbiome (which so many of us do).

Canned beans often contain BPA (bisphenol A), a hormone disruptor found in plastic bottles and cans that can wreck your health. BPA-free cans are a better choice, but they still contain other hormone disruptors like BPS and BPF. My recommendation is to buy dried beans and soak them overnight in water with a little salt. Cook your beans with a big strip of kombu (a seaweed) in a pressure cooker.

Another option is to add kombu, beans, and water to a large pot. Bring to a boil, and then reduce to a simmer for two to four hours. Drain your beans and use in any recipe. This helps reduce the gas-producing properties and makes them a lot easier to digest. If you have severe gut dysbiosis or an autoimmune disease, or are obese or diabetic, eliminate beans temporarily from your diet until your gut health and metabolism improve through following the Pegan Diet.

Soybeans generate the most confusion of any bean. Some believe soy causes breast cancer. Yet research points to their anti-angiogenic, cancer-preventive properties. And not all soy is the same. Avoid soy protein (found in fake meats, bars, and shakes), which is a chemically altered by-product of soybean oil production, often known as isolated soy protein or textured vegetable protein. Animal studies show it causes cancer, while whole traditional soy foods prevent cancer. Some worry about phytoestrogens (plant compounds called isoflavones, which bind to estrogen receptors) in soy. These can actually protect you from the effects of excess estrogen or xenoestrogens, the chemical toxins found in plastics like BPA and phthalates. Research shows that phytoestrogens can help with menopausal symptoms and prevent breast cancer.[13] Isoflavones protect us from cardiovascular disease, cognitive decline, and other age-related diseases.

Stay away from soybean oil and soy protein isolates. Stick with non-GMO, organic, traditional soybean foods like tofu, tempeh, miso, natto, and gluten-free soy sauce or tamari. These are processed in a way that makes them digestible and more beneficial. Tempeh, miso, and natto are also probiotic, gut-healthy foods.

GRAINS

Grains, in addition to beans, are a hot topic of debate between the Paleo and vegan crowds. Humans consumed no grains until about 10,000 years ago, so they are not an essential part of our diet. However, they have become a staple in our modern times, making up over 60 percent of our diet. Whole grains (not flours) can be a good source of fiber, phytonutrients, vitamins, minerals, essential fats, and even a little protein. On the other hand, large quantities of grains can be problematic for those with insulin resistance, irritable bowel, autoimmune disease, or inflammation—especially gluten-containing grains, including wheat, spelt, barley, rye, oats, farro, kamut, and triticale.

The gluten-free diet has become sexy, even if many have no clue why! The body reacts to gluten in various ways. Celiac disease affects 1 percent of the population, non-celiac gluten sensitivity affects about 20 percent of the population, and low-grade immune activation affects many more. When you eat gluten, your body produces the molecule *zonulin,* which creates a leaky gut by opening up the connections between intestinal cells. Normally these tight junctions are firmly stuck together like Legos to prevent food particles and other foreign particles from leaking into the spaces between cells. You do not want your intestinal lining to become leaky. It can create a cascade of damaging effects, including autoimmune disease and a host of inflammatory diseases. Today, scientists are confirming what we have suspected for a while: Most of us cannot properly process gluten.

Need a few more reasons to go easy on the gluten? The

new forms of hybridized wheat, known as dwarf wheat, contain amylopectin A, a super starch worse than sugar; many more inflammatory gliadin proteins that cause leaky gut; lots of the weed killer glyphosate; and lastly a preservative, calcium propionate, linked to mood, behavior, and attention problems and even autism. Makes you want to skip the breadbasket (I hope!).

I also want to touch on what I call "the new gluten," aka corn. Once gluten was identified as a villain, corn became a "health food fan" favorite. I don't mean corn on the cob, I mean corn flour, turned into tortillas, corn chips, gluten-free bread, and pasta. Ninety percent of corn grown in America is GMO doused with herbicides and pesticides. This is not ancient heirloom corn, grown by the Native Americans and full of medicinal compounds. Today's hybridized corn is bred for starch and sugar content, not nutrient density. The only thing dense in modern corn is the sugar content. If you're going to eat corn, I recommend non-GMO and ideally organic, and go easy on corn flour. Try heirloom corn products.

So, what kinds of grains should we eat? Not the ones that have been pulverized and turned into bread or baked products that cause blood sugar to spike more than regular table sugar. You read that right. Whole wheat bread is worse for you than plain old sugar. Flours of any kind in the form of bread, pasta, muffins, and pastries are the source of most metabolic disorders. For daily consumption, always choose whole grains like brown rice, red rice, wild rice, teff, amaranth, buckwheat, and quinoa (technically a seed).

Then there are the super grains. My favorite is black rice, also known as forbidden rice or the emperor's rice. It is full of phytonutrients and known as the blueberries of grains. My friend and mentor, Dr. Jeffrey Bland, is bringing Himalayan Tartary buckwheat into production in America. It is an ancient grain prized for being a rich source of powerful anti-inflammatory polyphenols, making it one of the most significant superfoods on the planet. Himalayan buckwheat polyphenols make up almost 90 percent of the antioxidant punch compared to 20 percent for regular buckwheat.[14] It contains many flavonoids, including rutin and quercetin. Quercetin has been promoted as one of the most powerful natural anti-inflammatories for COVID-19.

As with most foods, the dose of grains is key. I recommend ½ cup to 1 cup of grains per day. If you are an athlete and are metabolically healthy (only 12 percent of us), you may be able to include more grains.

IS WHITE RICE PEGAN-FRIENDLY?

I typically don't recommend white rice for individuals with belly fat and high blood sugar. Not many of us are metabolically healthy, and white rice can send your blood sugar on a roller-coaster ride. However, some can tolerate white rice in limited quantities without dramatic spikes in blood sugar. If you want to enjoy white rice, here's a way to make it super Pegan-friendly: After cooking the rice, allow it to cool in the fridge before eating it. This process turns the rice into resistant starch that is easier to digest and metabolize and feeds your good gut bacteria.

PRINCIPLE 4 TAKEAWAYS

1. **A handful or two of nuts and seeds every day is great.** Soak raw nuts overnight and lightly toast them to improve digestion. Snack on almonds, walnuts, cashews, macadamia nuts, hazelnuts, pecans, pumpkin seeds, chia seeds, hemp seeds, flaxseeds, pistachios, Brazil nuts, unsweetened nut butters, and nut milks with minimal ingredients and no added sugars.

2. **Eat non-starchy beans.** Lupini beans, lentils, peas or snow peas, black-eyed peas, mung beans, and traditional non-GMO and organic soy products are my favorites. The maximum serving is half a cup per day. Soak dried beans for a few hours or overnight or cook them with kombu in a pressure cooker or large pot. Avoid excessive amounts of kidney beans, lima beans, and baked beans, which are starchier.

3. **Stick to ½ to 1 cup of whole grains per day.** Avoid processed and refined grains. Eat them as whole kernels, not in some fake "whole grain" products like Whole Grain Cookie Crisp Cereal. If you have gut dysbiosis, weight problems, or autoimmune disease, take a three-week holiday from grains and notice how you feel. Many of my patients see an improvement in their symptoms and are able to lose weight when they come off grains temporarily.

Eat Your Meat as Medicine

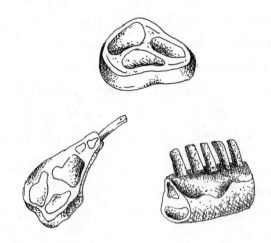

There are three primary considerations when it comes to the question of whether we should be eating meat:

1. Ethical and moral considerations
2. Environmental and climate impacts
3. Impacts on our health

The truth is more nuanced than meat, good or bad. While factory-farmed red meat is an environmental and climate catastrophe, is inhumane, and may have adverse health consequences, this is not true of meat from regeneratively raised animals. Is bison or wild elk the same as a feedlot steak for your health, the well-being of the animals, or the health of the environment? Absolutely not.

Regenerative agriculture applies a science-based approach that focuses on producing the highest-quality food while restoring ecosystems by building soil that sequesters carbon and holds tens of thousands of gallons of water per acre. This method of farming brings back pollinators, beneficial insects, and wildlife, and uses no or little chemical inputs (fertilizer, pesticides, and herbicides), while producing more nutrient-dense and abundant food. Regenerative farmers make up to 20 times more profit than their conventional neighbors. Globally, regenerative agriculture is recognized as critical to achieving food security, reversing climate change, restoring biodiversity, and improving health. The UN estimates if we converted 2 million of our 5 million hectares of degraded agricultural lands to regenerative farming, we could stop climate change for 20 years. The cost: $300 billion, or less than we spend annually on diabetes in America.

So the debate shouldn't be meat vs. plants. It should be regenerative agriculture vs. industrial agriculture. As Ross Conser, a regenerative farmer, said, "It's not the cow, it's the how."

MORAL AND ETHICAL CONSIDERATIONS

Religious, cultural, or ethical reasons may guide personal decisions about the consumption of animal products. I have monks and abbots as patients. I support them in building the healthiest possible diet without animal products. I understand the rationale for opposition to modern meat. Modern factory farms, or CAFOs (concentrated animal feeding operations), are an abomination. In 2020, Senators Cory

Booker and Elizabeth Warren introduced a bill to ban factory farming by 2040. The world is waking up to the horrors of industrial farming. In CAFOs, animals are fed unnatural diets of corn, soy, ground-up animal parts, chicken excrement, candy, antibiotics, and often hormones. Factory farming is a massive disaster for our environment, the climate, our health, the health of animals, farmworkers, workers in processing plants, and everyone and everything in between. If you want to do anything to create a healthier world, stop eating factory-farmed meat now.

However, all industrial farming, whether we are raising animals or growing fruits and vegetables, is inherently destructive—tillage leading to soil erosion and heavy use of fertilizers, pesticides, and herbicides is harmful to flora and fauna. Even industrial organic plant agriculture destroys natural habitats. Studies estimate that 7 billion animals die each year from plant agriculture—rodents, rabbits, birds, and insects. Over the last 50 years, we have lost 50 percent of our birds from industrial agriculture. While regenerative agriculture can increase the health of ecosystems and biodiversity, there is always some death involved in creating life, directly or indirectly. Is the life of a rabbit that dies in a cabbage patch worth less than that of a chicken or cow on a factory farm? Like it or not, most of our plant and animal agriculture today is destructive. If you're vegan for ethical reasons, I implore you to consider advocating for regenerative farming to prevent all of the unnecessary harm that occurs during industrial farming. In Principle 14, we'll talk more about how to be a healthy vegan while eating the Pegan diet.

ENVIRONMENTAL AND CLIMATE CONSIDERATIONS

In addition to animal welfare, the environment and the climate also drive dietary choices. The Intergovernmental Panel on Climate Change (IPCC) estimates that 14.5 percent of greenhouse gases are due to livestock production on factory farms. Of that, 9.5 percent results from the production of feed for feedlots and from processing and transportation. Only 5 percent is from methane produced by livestock. To put that in perspective, the amount of methane produced by rotting vegetables in landfills accounts for 16 percent of global methane production, more than 3 times that produced by livestock. Rice paddies produce 3 percent of global methane. And while methane is 25 times more potent a greenhouse gas than carbon dioxide, it is short-lived in the atmosphere, unlike carbon dioxide. The amount of methane in the atmosphere today is about the same as it was 12,000 years ago, before fossil fuels and agriculture.

Modern agriculture is also fertilizer-intensive. Four hundred billion pounds of nitrogen-based fertilizer are used globally every year, representing a major source of greenhouse gas emissions. Fertilizer production accounts for about 2 percent of total global energy use. Most of this comes from fracking, which produces about a quarter of all methane released into the atmosphere. Nitrous oxide, the result of nitrogen-based fertilizer, is 300 times more potent a greenhouse gas than CO_2, destroys the organic matter (carbon) in the soil, and runs off into rivers, lakes, and streams, killing millions of tons of nutritious seafood worldwide. Instead of buying fertilizer, with all its downstream consequences, farmers can make their own. Animals integrated into farming systems have been the main source of fertilizer for thousands of years. Taking animals out of integrated ecological agricultural systems and piling them into feedlots has been an unmitigated disaster for the earth, the climate, and yes, us humans too.

It was the 168 million ruminants roaming North America (bison, elk, antelope, deer, etc., compared to 95 million beef cattle in the United States today) that built 8 to 50 feet of rich topsoil. We have lost one-third of that topsoil and are projected to lose all of it in sixty harvests. Globally, soil carbon loss accounts for one-third of the 1 trillion tons of carbon in the atmosphere. Integrating animals into a diverse regenerative farm ecosystem is essential to building soil and restoring ecosystems. You may choose to eat them or not, but they are a critical part of regenerative farming. Regenerative livestock production converts more than 432 billion kilograms of food inedible for humans, from land not suitable for growing crops, into nutrient-dense, high-quality protein, and produces 4 billion kilograms of fertilizer (poop) in the process. The side effect? Reducing net greenhouse gas emissions (GHGE) by 86 percent, making regenerative livestock production 74 percent lower in GHGE than the cultivation of commodity crops used for feed or even plant-based meats like processed soy burgers (Impossible Burger).[15] Sadly, today, regenerative practices make up less than 1 percent of agricultural production. However, regenerative livestock practices are scalable and can replace factory farming globally. Ruminants foraging on diverse plants containing phytochemicals such as saponins and tannins dramatically reduce methane production.[16] Regenerative practices that build soil microbiology create lots of methanotrophic bacteria (bugs that suck methane out of the air and put it into the soil). Feeding cows seaweed also lowers their methane production! When raised regeneratively, animals are a carbon sink, not a carbon source, even after accounting for all the inputs and cow burps and methane emissions.

Of the eighty science-based methods to mitigate climate change documented by Project Drawdown (an organization that identifies the world's most effective ways to draw down carbon from the atmosphere), regenerative agricultural practices were collectively the number one solution to suck carbon out of the atmosphere and reverse climate change.

IS MEAT HEALTHY OR HARMFUL?

This, my friends, is the real question. Ending factory farming and scaling up regenerative agriculture addresses most of the concerns about climate, environment, and inhumane treatment of animals, but the key question is, will meat kill you, or is it a nutrient-dense health food?

Go into the National Library of Medicine research database. You will find (as of May 2020) 100,333 studies on meat. You can find studies showing anything you want. Meat is the devil. Meat is a superfood. Why? Nutritional research is tough. Most studies examine the dietary patterns of large populations over long periods and look for correlations. However, there are so many confounding factors that it is hard to know what's causing what. If people who eat meat also eat a highly processed diet full of junk food and sugar, and low in fruits and veggies, their disease and death risks are higher. If they eat meat as part of a whole food diet, their risk of disease goes down. In a 2019 review of sixty-one studies of 4 million people, including many randomized controlled trials, researchers found no link between meat and disease or death.[17] And those studies were conducted on conventional feedlot meat, not regenerative or grass-finished meat, which may have beneficial health effects.

Not all food is the same. Eat a flavorless cardboard-tasting tomato grown in a greenhouse. Then try a ripe, juicy organic heirloom tomato picked from the vine in your garden on a warm late August day. Both are tomatoes, but they couldn't be more different in terms of taste, nutrient density, and phytonutrient content. Now imagine a wild elk, or even a regeneratively raised cow, foraging on phytonutrient-rich, omega-3-dense plants. How does that compare to a feedlot cow, fed an unnatural diet and pumped full of growth hormones and antibiotics? If food is information, how could they be the same? Yet most studies don't distinguish. Are the participants in these studies eating conventional meat, which might not have any effect on death or disease? Are they eating processed meat along with a processed food diet, which has been shown to cause cancer? Or are they eating grass-fed meat in the context of a real, whole foods diet, which might actually benefit health?

Quality matters, and what you eat with your meat matters too. A whole foods, nutrient-dense, high-fiber, prebiotic- and probiotic-rich, phytonutrient-rich diet — or a burger, fries, and Coke — makes all the difference. Preparation also matters. High-temperature cooking or grilling (veggies or meat) produces toxic compounds, including heterocyclic amines, polycyclic aromatic hydrocarbons, and advanced glycation end products (AGEs), which can damage your arteries and cause cancer. I also recommend cooking your meat with spices. The Maasai people of Africa eat only milk and meat, but they add twelve spices to their milk and twenty-eight spices to their meat, preventing the production of harmful compounds that can occur during cooking. In Morocco, cancer rates are low despite heavy meat intake. The slow cooking of meat with dozens of antioxidant and anti-inflammatory spices is protective. Studies show dramatic reductions in oxidative stress markers when meat is consumed with herbs, spices, and polyphenols, such as red wine, olive oil, and balsamic vinegar.[18]

Striking new research has found a rich array of phytonutrients in grass-fed meat. Disease-preventing and health-promoting medicinal plant chemicals in meat? How is that possible? You are not what you eat; you are whatever you are eating has eaten. As outlined in a remarkable paper titled "Health Promoting Compounds Are Higher in Grass-Fed Meat and Milk," published in *Frontiers in Nutrition,* scientists from Duke University found healing phytochemicals in grass-fed meat, such as terpenoids, phenols, carotenoids, and antioxidants with anti-inflammatory, anti-carcinogenic, and cardioprotective effects. While we know about improved profiles in grass-fed meat of fatty acids, omega-3 fats, anticancer metabolism-boosting fat called CLA, and higher levels of minerals and vitamins, the discovery of phytochemicals in meat is new ground. Cows raised in feedlots have limited diets of silage, mostly corn. Regeneratively raised cows, as opposed to just grass-fed ones, may eat dozens and dozens of different plant species as they forage. Each plant contains different phytochemicals, antioxidants, vitamins, and minerals. Different plants extract different nutrients from the soil. For example, foraging grass-fed dairy cows have up to 23 times more powerful anti-cancer, antiviral, antioxidant, anti-inflammatory compounds called monoterpenes compared to conventional dairy cows.

Goats raised on pasture have the same amount of phenolic compounds as green tea, one of the most important superfoods on the planet! Quercetin, found in onions and helpful against viruses, and caffeic acid, found in coffee and anti-inflammatory, are both high in goats that forage on diverse shrubs and grasses. This is game-changing information.

What about saturated fat and blood cholesterol? Turns out the main saturated fat in meat, stearic acid, is neutral when it comes to blood cholesterol. The "saturated fat is bad" dogma is not so simple, as I explained in my book *Eat Fat, Get Thin*. There are many types of saturated fat, all with different properties. Fat in regeneratively raised grass-fed meat is different from fat in corn-fed meat. According to the American Heart Association, we should limit saturated fat to less than 5 percent of our calories. No more breast milk for babies, then? Breast milk is 25 percent saturated fat. And your genes may affect your body's response to saturated fat (more on that in Principle 7). Some patients' lipids dramatically improve on a high–saturated fat diet; others worsen. There are genetic tests that can help determine how you might respond. The best way to find out? Experiment on yourself. Test your numbers. It turns out cholesterol is far more complicated than just total, LDL, or HDL. The size and number of the cholesterol particles matter. The only way to get an accurate picture is to measure your cholesterol profile with an NMR test (LabCorp) or Cardio IQ (Quest Diagnostics). Ask your doctor for these tests. They are not what doctors typically order. It turns out that the sugar and starch in your diet cause the damaging type of lipid profile, with small HDL particles, small LDL particles, and high triglycerides. You should worry more about the impact of sugar and starch on your cholesterol than the impact of grass-fed beef.

HOW CAN I REALISTICALLY AFFORD GRASS-FED, ORGANIC MEAT?

I know it can be hard to find quality meat. There are a few great options out there. One option is to participate in a cow share from a regenerative farm. At Mariposa Ranch, you can get grass-fed meat for an average of about $8 per pound, which is pretty good. I've seen more and more affordable ways to get grass-fed organic meat at places like Whole Foods as well. Here are my favorite online sources for buying quality affordable meat.

- Thrivemarket.com
- Butcherbox.com
- Mariposaranchmeat.com
- Grassrootscoop.com

PRINCIPLE 5 TAKEAWAYS

1. **Meat can be a health food.** After decades of reviewing the science, it is clear that grass-fed, regeneratively raised meat, cooked in the right way and combined with medicinal spices in the context of a plant-rich, whole foods, unprocessed diet,

is not only not bad for your health—it might be beneficial, providing the most nutrient-dense protein available, rich in omega-3 fats, phytochemicals, antioxidants, and bioavailable forms of vitamins and minerals. Quality is vital in every aspect of eating, and especially with meat.

2. **Meat should not be the star of the show.** While we need the right amount of protein for our age and activity level (ranging from a minimum 0.8 grams/kg to 1.6 grams/kg or more for certain athletes), the Pegan Diet is not a high-protein diet. Its mainstay is plants. Meat is the side dish.

3. **Mix up your diet with plant and animal proteins.** Eat a palm-sized piece of protein (either grass-fed meats, poultry, eggs, or fish) twice a day. This rule works whether you are a 6'10" basketball player or a five-year-old.

4. **Avoid high-temperature cooking, grilling, frying, smoking, or charring.** Instead, focus on low-temperature methods of cooking like baking, roasting, and poaching. Use a lot of spices, and eat wild and regenerative foods when possible.

Be Picky About Poultry, Eggs, and Fish

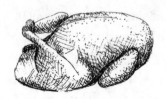

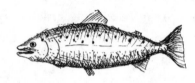

Industrial poultry and fish farming are destructive to animals, humans, and the planet. These foods make up a large part of the human diet worldwide. We have to be picky when choosing fish, poultry, and eggs. Our health and the health of the planet demand it.

CHOOSING POULTRY AND EGGS

Conventional chickens are pumped full of corn and antibiotics, making them fatter than ever and their meat less nutritious than ever. Birds raised in concentrated animal feeding operations (CAFOs) live in horrendous conditions—small cages, with little access to the outside world. Because of the unsanitary conditions, they are more likely to carry dangerous pathogens like Salmonella and *E. coli*. Workers in chicken factories also struggle under terrible working conditions. Bathroom breaks are so rare that some employees in chicken processing plants have reported having to wear diapers. The toxic waste produced by Tyson from its poultry factories is second only to waste produced by steel factories in environmental pollution. The key takeaway is to avoid conventionally raised chicken for your sake and for the sake of the food workers, the chickens, and the environment.

While beef labeling is mostly straightforward—feedlot, hormone-free, antibiotic-free, grass-fed, and regenerative—chicken labeling is a confusing free-for-all. The choice isn't as simple as organic or conventional; there's free-range, pasture-raised, cage-free, vegetarian-fed, grain-fed, antibiotic-free, hormone-free, all-natural, and so on. You've likely encountered all of these befuddling labels designed to make us believe that we're making the best choice for the chickens and for our bodies. In reality, most of these labels are meaningless. The label "all-natural" on any food product typically means anything but. If you see vegetarian-fed or grain-fed poultry or eggs, turn the other way. Chickens are not vegetarians; they roam on the pasture eating worms and other bugs. Free-range implies that the birds are free to enjoy the outdoors, but this label does not require any designated amount of time that the birds can roam, and it does not tell us about the birds' diet. In an ideal world, pasture-raised poultry and eggs are best; these birds freely roam around and eat their natural diet. For now, they are hard to find (it's a bit easier to find pasture-raised eggs); but if you can't find pasture-raised, go for organic. This at least guarantees that the bird was not pumped with antibiotics or fed grains sprayed with pesticides. Organic birds often have more access to the outdoors.

As for the effects of poultry on our health? Poultry is leaner than most red meat, but it still contains saturated fat (albeit slightly less). It also contains monounsaturated fats like palmitoleic acid, which is a powerful infection-fighting antimicrobial fat. Think chicken soup for colds and the flu! As we learned in the previous principle, we don't have to fear these fats, especially when eating a low-glycemic diet, limited in starches and sugars.

What about eggs? The main concern here is cholesterol, but the misinformation on the effects of dietary cholesterol is finally coming to the surface. We now understand that some of the foods we were told to avoid for years are among the most beneficial. Eggs are actually a superfood. The yolk is the most nutritious part—low in calories, high in protein, and full of vitamins, minerals, antioxidants, choline, and phyto-nutrients (yes, the yolk has carotenoids like lutein). After all, egg yolks contain all the nutrients needed for creating a whole new life. Ditch those egg white omelets. Whole egg omelets taste better anyway! There is one caveat: Some people are sensitive to eggs. If you have an autoimmune condition or suspect an egg sensitivity, eliminate eggs for three weeks. Add them back in on day 22 and see how your body responds. You might need to stay off eggs for a few months or more.

CHOOSING FISH AND SEAFOOD

When it comes to fish, there are two main concerns. First, we have polluted the oceans, and many fish are full of mercury, microplastics, PCBs, and other contaminants. And second, our fishing practices result in overfishing and depletion of whole fish populations, such as Atlantic cod. According to my friend Paul Greenberg, a fisherman and fish researcher, 30 percent of commercial fish stocks are overfished. Industrial crops of corn and wheat are reliant on nitrogen fertilizer (400 billion pounds a year globally), which runs off into rivers and oceans, causing algal blooms that suck all the oxygen from the water, leaving lakes, rivers, and oceans lifeless. There are 400 coastal dead zones worldwide the size of Europe, on which 500 billion people depend for food. The Mississippi River drains the great agricultural lands of the Midwest into the Gulf of Mexico, causing a dead zone the size of New Jersey that kills 212,000 metric tons of fish a year. In other words, fish and seafood, nutritional superfoods, have to die so we can grow corn and soy for factory-farmed meat.

Farmed fish comes with a whole set of concerns—more omega-6 and fewer omega-3 fats from soy and grain feed, antibiotics because of overcrowding, higher levels of PCBs, lower levels of protein, and the need to use 5 to 10 pounds of fish chow harvested from the oceans to make 1 pound of fish humans want to eat. Luckily, there's a way to choose fish that is rich in nutrients and low in toxins—specifically, wild-caught and sustainably harvested farm-raised fish.

My biggest piece of advice is to eat fish that are lower in mercury. I know Americans love their tuna, but the bigger the fish, the more likely you are to be exposed to things like mercury and microplastics. Smaller fish like anchovies and sardines are loaded with nutrients and less likely to contain toxins. If you're grossed out by either of those, I've included a few recipes in this book that will dazzle the whole family. Check out the Simple Arrabbiata Sauce on page 229.

In addition to anchovies and sardines, I recommend salmon, mackerel, and herring (with sardines, often referred to as SMASH fish). They are rich in omega-3 fats, and they're less likely to contain high levels of mercury. If you're worried about mercury, get your levels tested by a functional medicine doctor. Also, get your omega-3 levels checked to see if you need to incorporate more fish or perhaps a fish oil or omega-3 supplement.

Regenerative ocean farming is a growing movement. Mixed aquacultures of seaweed, scallops, oysters, mussels, and clams require zero inputs (fertilizers, cleaning agents, additives, feedstuffs) while sequestering carbon (think of seaweed as underwater rainforests). The seaweed can be eaten or turned into bioplastics, animal feed, fertilizer, and more. Using seaweed for compost and fertilizer creates a virtuous nutrient loop where carbon, nitrogen, and phosphorus are upcycled or reused, thereby enriching soil and increasing crop yields. Growing seaweed in just 3.8 percent of the ocean off the coast of California could completely offset all of California's agricultural emissions. Feeding cattle seaweed can reduce their methane emissions by 60 percent. One nonprofit, GreenWave, helps ocean farmers learn the methods and get started with very little investment. This is the future!

PRINCIPLE 6 TAKEAWAYS

1. **Eat pasture-raised chicken, turkey, duck, and eggs when possible.** Organic is the next-best thing. Switch up your proteins. I recommend two 4-ounce servings a day of animal protein. Another way to think about this is a palm-sized piece of meat or protein per meal. I typically recommend eating eggs two to three times a week. Some people feel great eating eggs more often. I like to switch up breakfasts to get in a variety of plant foods. Some days I'll have a smoothie, some days I'll have bulletproof coffee, and other days I'll have an omelet with a side of greens. For quality chicken, check out thrivemarket.com, butcherbox.com, grassrootscoop.com, localharvest.org (poultry and eggs), and eatwild.com.

2. **Stick with low-mercury fish, three times a week.** Eat wild fish and seafood. My favorites are wild salmon, either canned or fresh, and small, low-toxin fish like sardines, anchovies, herring, and mackerel. For seafood, I recommend clams, mussels, oysters, shrimp, and scallops. When you can't find wild fish, eat fish farmed with sustainable, restorative, or regenerative practices. Check out cleanfish.com to learn more. Fishwise.org is also a useful resource for sustainable fish in your area. Stay away from toxic or endangered fish. Look for the Global Aquaculture Alliance Best Practices symbol. Seafood Watch also recommends different eco-certification organizations for farmed and wild-caught seafood, such as Aquaculture Stewardship. My other favorite resources for quality fish include vitalchoice.com, thrivemarket.com, and butcherbox.com. They have wild and sustainably farmed seafood.

PRINCIPLE 7

Have Fats with Every Meal

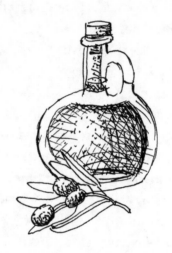

Fat has been unfairly vilified for decades. It clogs your arteries and makes you fat, they said. It has more than twice the calories per gram compared to carbs and protein, we were warned. We all followed the low-fat advice provided by experts and our government for the last 40 years. What happened? We got fat and diabetic—big-time. Obesity rates have gone from 5 percent to 42 percent since I was born (that's an 800 percent increase). When I started eating fats with every meal, I became happier, stronger, and more energized. The right fats can make you healthy and lean, and can fuel your brain. The wrong fats can be deadly. Unlike sugar, which is pretty much all bad, fats are complicated.

The Pegan Diet respects and honors that we are all

different—genetically, metabolically, and culturally. What is medicine to one may be poison to another. Some people thrive on a high-fat diet (cholesterol plummets, waistlines shrink, diabetes disappears, and even heart failure risk improves). Others gain weight and struggle with abnormal cholesterol. The best way to know how different foods might impact your body is to experiment and test. Your body knows. Listen to it! No dogma or study will tell you what works for you. Roger Williams, the father of biochemical individuality (the idea that we are all genetically and biologically unique), once said: "Statistical humans are of little interest. I am interested in real humans." Me too.

OMEGA-6 VS. OMEGA-3 FATS: WHAT WE KNOW

While a few low-fat evangelists still warn about the dangers of avocados, nuts, and olive oil, their advice contradicts an overwhelming body of evidence on these protective foods. Certain fats are essential for life. Whole foods containing mostly monounsaturated fats—olive oil, nuts and seeds, and avocados—help prevent heart disease, lower blood pressure, and improve insulin sensitivity. Polyunsaturated fats include omega-3 and omega-6 fatty acids, which are key building blocks for life. Our bodies can't make these fats, so we have to consume them, and maintaining a healthy ratio between these fats is also critical. While debate rages on the pros and cons of refined plant-based oils (soybean, canola, safflower, grape-seed, etc.), there is no debate on eating omega-6 fats from whole foods such as beans, grains, and nuts and seeds. They are safe as long as you are getting enough omega-3 fats. The problem is that the Western diet contains far too many omega-6 fats from the wrong sources, like GMO soybean oil (10 percent of our calories, mostly from processed foods) and GMO canola oil, and too few omega-3 fats from fish; pasture-raised eggs; flax, chia, and hemp seeds; and grass-fed meat. Polyunsaturated omega-6 fats are healthful, but stick to whole food forms found in beans, grains, nuts, and seeds. Cold-pressed, unrefined non-GMO oils, including sesame and high oleic sunflower oil, can be used occasionally. Stay away from all industrially processed, heat- and solvent-extracted, oxidized oils. My favorite oils for cooking at high temperatures are avocado oil, coconut oil, and ghee. They all have high smoke points. For low-heat cooking (like tomato sauce), I like olive oil. On salads, and for drizzling, I like almond oil, macadamia oil, sesame seed oil, tahini, flax oil, hemp oil, and, of course, extra virgin olive oil.

SATURATED FAT: HEALTHY OR HARMFUL?

Saturated fats are found in dairy, meat, coconut oil, and even many plant foods, including healthful nuts, olives, and avocados. Even heart-healthy olive oil is 20 percent saturated fat. Medical and government advice has vilified saturated fat. We have been told it is the number one cause of heart disease. But saturated fat may not be the villain we once believed it to be.

There is no single, notoriously bad saturated fat except the recently banned trans fats, which are plant-based oils chemically altered to make them solid—think shortening!

There are many saturated fats that have different effects on the body. What you eat with these fats is what matters. Butter in your cookies may be deadly, while butter on your veggies may be healthful. Key take-home: Do not eat saturated fats in combination with starch and sugar (which unfortunately is how most people consume them); that causes inflammation, weight gain, diabetes, dementia, and heart disease.

Individual genetic and biological differences also significantly impact responses to dietary saturated fats. Data on saturated fats are mixed and confusing (as is most nutrition science). For most of us, including a little grass-fed butter or other dairy, meat, or even some unrefined coconut oil is fine. The key again is to see what works for you. One patient on a ketogenic (high-fat, low-carb) diet with loads of butter and coconut oil dropped her total cholesterol by 100 points, her triglycerides by 200 points, and raised her HDL cholesterol by 30 points. She also lost 20 stubborn pounds. Another thin bike racer's lipids turn scary on a high–saturated fat diet. Be your own guinea pig. Try, test, and try again.

In functional medicine, we don't look at just your total, LDL, and HDL cholesterol. Why? High cholesterol alone is not as problematic as once believed. It's the overall pattern and quality of your cholesterol profile and your other risk factors that matter most. We look at a particular test that measures the quality of your lipids—the particle size and number. Do you have large, fluffy, protective LDL particles? Or do you have small, dense, dangerous heart disease–causing LDL particles? This test is called the NMR particle-size test from LabCorp (or Cardio IQ from Quest

Diagnostics). Without the right tests, you are flying blind in trying to assess your risk for heart disease. If you're on a high-fat, low-carb diet and your cholesterol keeps going up, test your particle size. If you have lots of small, dense particles, a high-fat diet is not the one for you. See the Resources section on page 245 for more information on how to get and interpret this test.

Nutritional genetic tests can also help guide your dietary choices. Your inability to tolerate saturated fats might be entirely genetic, and having that information is critical. For example, patients with the *APOE4* gene, which can increase the risk of heart disease and Alzheimer's disease, are prone to inflammation, and they don't do well with a lot of saturated fat. They should limit saturated fat but enjoy fats from fish, olive oil, avocados, nuts, and seeds. In my practice, I use nutritional genetic testing to help solve challenging clinical problems and personalize diets for my patients. We'll talk about this more in Principle 12.

WHAT FAT TO EAT

Bottom line: Even though fats are complicated, eating a fat-free diet is not good for your health. We need fats to survive. Every cell is made of fat; our nerve coverings are made of fat; our brain is mostly fat; our hormones are made of fat; our cells and metabolism run better on fat. Fats help you absorb all of the beneficial fat-soluble vitamins in plant foods, and some fats have been shown to reduce the risk of heart disease, type 2 diabetes, and obesity. The key is to eat the right fats and stay clear of the wrong fats. Here's a cheat sheet that will make it really simple.

Eat	Avoid or Limit
Organic extra virgin olive oil	Soybean oil
Organic avocado oil	Canola oil
Walnut oil	Corn oil
Almond oil	Safflower oil
Macadamia oil	Sunflower oil
Unrefined sesame oil	Peanut oil
Tahini (sesame seed paste)	Vegetable oil, grape-seed oil
Flax oil	Vegetable shortening
Hemp oil	Margarine and butter substitutes
Avocado, olives, and other plant sources of fat	Anything that says "hydrogenated"
Nuts and seeds	
Butter from pastured, grass-fed cows or goats	
Grass-fed ghee	
Organic, humanely raised tallow, lard, duck fat, or chicken fat	
Coconut oil or MCT oil (medium-chain triglycerides)	
Sustainable palm oil (look for certified sustainable palm oil)	

PRINCIPLE 7 TAKEAWAY

Don't fear fat; instead, eat the right fats with every meal. Fat won't make you fat, unless you eat it with starch and sugar like most Americans. Eat 3 to 5 servings of fat per day, and eat fats mostly with vegetables. Unless it is trans fat, it won't cause heart disease. My favorite fats are avocados, olives, nuts and seeds, and traditional oils like extra virgin olive oil and avocado oil. Small amounts of butter, grass-fed ghee, and coconut or MCT oil are fine for most of us. If you're eating a high-fat diet and are curious about how it's affecting your body, I recommend looking into the NMR particle-size cholesterol test.

PRINCIPLE 8

Avoid Dairy (Mostly)

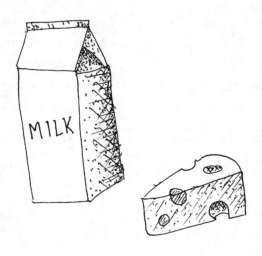

Milk. It does a body good by building strong, healthy bones. Or does it? Our American love affair with milk has more to do with good PR and marketing ("Got Milk?") than good science. Milk and dairy sensitivities are among the biggest causes of symptoms that I see in my practice. If milk isn't the health food we've been told it is, why do our own government's dietary guidelines implore us to consume three glasses of milk a day? Certainly not for scientific reasons, according to two of the world's leading nutrition scientists, Harvard's David Ludwig and Walter Willett, who reviewed 100 of the top studies on milk for an article in the *New England Journal of Medicine*.[19] The title should have been "Got Proof?" Apparently not. In fact, while the purported benefits turn out to be untrue, there are very real risks for cancer, allergies, autoimmune disease, hormone disorders, eczema, and digestive problems, not to mention the environmental and climate harms from factory-farmed dairy.

THE CALCIUM MYTH

We were told that the biggest reason we needed dairy is that it's the best source of calcium and will give us strong bones and reduce fractures. Oops. We got that wrong—dead wrong. Besides the fact that countries with the highest dairy intake, like Sweden, have the highest fracture rates, and countries with the lowest intake, like China and Indonesia, have the lowest fracture rates, a study of 100,000 men found that one glass of milk a day consumed as an adolescent increased fracture risk by 9 percent,[20] and each additional glass of milk increased the risk of broken bones by another 9 percent.

How else, you might wonder, will you get your calcium and vitamin D? First, milk is fortified with vitamin D—it is not naturally found in dairy. The best natural sources of vitamin D are herring, porcini mushrooms, and sunlight. Where do cows get their calcium? From plants. Why eat secondhand calcium when you can get it firsthand from greens (kale, collards, arugula), tofu, sesame seeds (especially tahini), chia seeds, sardines, and canned salmon with bones?

THE LOW-FAT MYTH

I'm sure you've heard that low-fat dairy will help you lose weight. That's also incorrect. Kids, adolescents, and adults who consume low-fat milk gain more weight. Why? Fat makes you full, so you eat less overall. It turns out that full-fat, not low-fat, dairy may reduce the risk of diabetes.[21] These findings are based on measuring actual dairy fat levels in the blood, not just using food questionnaires. A 22-year study of 3,000 seniors examined the link between dairy intake, heart disease, and death.[22] Individuals who had higher blood levels of saturated fatty acids from dairy had a 42 percent lower risk of death from stroke and no increased heart disease risk. The researchers suggested that the current dietary guidelines be reevaluated to stop recommending reduced-fat dairy options.

Even though whole, full-fat dairy is a better choice than skim and low-fat, I typically never recommend traditional cow milk products. Up to 70 percent of the world's population is lactose intolerant. Most of my patients feel better without milk and cheese in their diet. They report improvements in skin and digestion. They feel less congested. It turns out milk is nature's perfect food, but only if you are a calf.

Milk also increases insulin-like growth factor 1 (IGF-1) in humans, which is like Miracle-Gro for cancer cells. Not only does milk fail the science tests for health benefits, but also modern industrial cow dairy makes many people very sick.

IF YOU WANT DAIRY, HERE'S SOME ADVICE

There are a few dairy products that I include occasionally and recommend to my patients. If you love dairy, try sheep or goat (or some heirloom cow) products, which have less inflammatory and better-tolerated A2 casein. Most cows today have high levels of the protein A1 casein, which causes inflammation, allergies, acne, eczema, and more. A2 milk contains glutathione, a powerful natural antioxidant, anti-inflammatory, detoxifying compound. If you like only cow dairy, my recommendation is to choose grass-fed, full-fat dairy, ideally regeneratively raised, and sourced from A2 cows. Go to a2milk.com to find sources near you. Guernsey and Jersey cows produce more A2 milk, as do most Indian and African cows.

I personally eat grass-fed ghee and butter, grass-fed sheep yogurt, or goat or sheep cheese (from animals raised on their traditional diets). Butter is a rich source of butyrate, a fatty acid that can prevent cancer, speed up your metabolism, and reduce inflammation. Ghee (a traditional Indian form of butter with casein and whey removed) is a lot easier for people to digest, and it's great for higher-temperature cooking. Probiotic-rich kefir and yogurt have some benefits, and, along with goat and sheep dairy, they are typically the only forms of dairy I recommend for patients who have gut imbalances. Stick to forms without all of the sugar. Many "fruit-sweetened" yogurts have more sugar per ounce than a can of soda! You can add your own berries at home.

Here's a cheat sheet for choosing dairy.

Eat	Avoid or Limit
Grass-fed, full-fat unsweetened yogurt	All dairy if you have allergies, acne, digestive issues, or an autoimmune disease
Kefir (fermented cow milk)	Dairy from conventionally raised cows
Grass-fed butter or ghee	Skim milk, low-fat, or nonfat dairy products
Goat and sheep dairy if not dairy-sensitive	Cheese made from skim milk or reduced-fat milk

PRINCIPLE 8 TAKEAWAY

Dairy is not an essential food group. It is likely harmful for most people. Do not consume low-fat or reduced-fat dairy products. They typically contain sugar and additives and may increase weight gain. Is a glass of milk better than soda? Yes. But that's not saying much. If you love dairy, choose grass-fed heirloom A2 cow dairy or goat or sheep dairy. Grass-fed butter, ghee, and unsweetened grass-fed sheep and goat yogurt, kefir, and cheese are fine from time to time if you tolerate dairy. If you're lactose intolerant, sensitive to dairy, or have digestive issues, avoid dairy completely.

Eat Like a Regenetarian

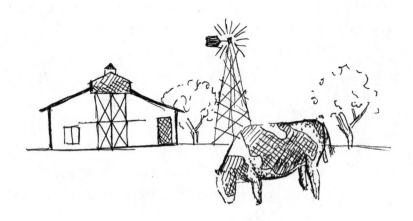

Our agriculture system is destructive—for the earth and for human health. The way we produce food destroys soil, mows down rainforests, depletes our freshwater resources, and drives massive loss of biodiversity. (We have lost 75 percent of our pollinator species, 90 percent of our edible plant species, and half of all livestock species, not to mention millions of other species of flora and fauna.) The food produced by industrial agriculture leads to at least 11 million deaths a year and drives our obesity epidemic. We need to build a regenerative system—one that regenerates the earth and human health. The good news is that it's more possible than ever.

OUR DEPLETED PLANET

In my last book, *Food Fix,* I mapped this all out, including how the food system is the number one contributor to climate change, and how fixing it is our number one solution. If you are not worried about climate change, you should be concerned about this: The UN estimates we have only sixty harvests left before we run out of soil. Why is this important? If you have (or plan to have) children or grandchildren, they will need to eat. No soil. No food. No humans. Aside from driving climate change and soil loss, our modern farming practices destroy natural resources and biodiversity, kill coral reefs, pollute oceans, destroy rainforests, and will ultimately lead to massive food insecurity. Our very way of growing food is threatening our future ability to grow food.

Our food system is responsible for almost half of all greenhouse gas emissions—from deforestation, destructive agricultural practices, food waste, and soil loss and damage. The soil loss accounts for one-third of all the carbon now in the atmosphere, or 300 billion tons of CO_2. One-fifth of fossil fuels are used for our food system, which is more than for transportation by planes, ships, cars, and trucks combined.

What we do to the planet we do to our bodies, and what we do to our bodies we do to the planet. Like it or not, we humans are part of the biological ecosystem. Scientists have coined a new term to describe our epoch (like the Ice Age, for example)—the *Anthropocene,* reflecting the first time in history that humans are the main factor driving changes to global climates and ecosystems.

As a doctor, I realized that I could not cure chronic diseases like obesity, diabetes, and heart disease in my office. The solution is on the farm and in our grocery stores, kitchens, and restaurants—in other words, in our food system. Food is medicine for humans. And food, grown in ways that are restorative and regenerative, is medicine for the planet.

The belief held by many is that a regenerative, climate-friendly diet is a plant-based vegan diet. Yes, we should all be eating a plant-rich diet for our health. Factory farms are an unmitigated environmental and climate disaster and should be banned, but this doesn't mean that animals should be banned from agriculture.

The science is clear. Animals *must* be included in the natural cycle of regenerative agriculture to build soil, produce fertilizer, conserve water, and eliminate the need for toxic agricultural chemicals. Eating them is optional. Integrating them into diverse natural farm ecosystems is not. A vegan vs. an omnivore diet is a false choice for the environment and climate. We can eat all the plant-based soy burgers we want, but it will not save us from climate change.

HOW DOES REGENERATIVE AGRICULTURE WORK?

Regeneratively raised animals are a net benefit to climate change by restoring the largest carbon sink on the planet, far greater than all the rainforests, a sink that can store 3 times as much carbon as exists today in the atmosphere: soil. There is no better carbon capture technology on the planet than photosynthesis. It's free and exists nearly everywhere. The best way to build soil, by far, is to mimic natural grassland animals' behavior with managed grazing.

Overgrazing is destructive and leads to increasing desertification. (We lose the equivalent of Nicaragua in arable land every year to desert.) Forty percent of agricultural land is not suitable for growing crops but is perfect for managed grazing and regenerative agriculture. Some estimate we could draw down 50 to 100 percent of all carbon released in the atmosphere since the industrial revolution if we scaled up regenerative agriculture.

The side effects of regenerative agriculture are all good ones: It produces far more nutrient-dense food, restores nutrient-rich soil, and restores natural habitats for insects, birds, and mammals. The animals (cows, chickens, pigs, sheep, goats) naturally seek out plants with the most phytonutrients, minerals, vitamins, and medicinal compounds while being raised in the most humane way possible. Right now, regenerative farms account for only 1 percent of agriculture. The siren cry of big agriculture is that while organic, local, and regenerative farming is nice, it will not feed the world. This view has been debunked. Globally, scientists, governments, and the UN understand the urgent need for a new approach to growing food—for both our health and the planet's health.

Regenerative agriculture is more profitable for farmers (up to 20 times more profitable) in a world where the average farmer, forced into bank loans and crop insurance, and buying seeds and chemicals from Big Ag companies, loses about $1,600 a year. It also produces higher yields and better-quality food. When we vote with our dollars and our forks by choosing regeneratively grown food, we send a message to Big Food that we want more sustainable farms. Companies like General Mills, Nestlé, Danone, and more are investing in regenerative agriculture. Some food companies are even paying farmers to convert to regenerative agriculture, stepping in where the government has not because they understand their supply chain of raw materials from agriculture is threatened if our current farming practices continue unchecked.

YOUR CHOICES MATTER

Eating for a healthy planet isn't just about big companies and policies. Your everyday choices are just as impactful. Food waste, lack of proper recycling, and overuse of plastic contributes to climate change. In fact, food waste is one of the biggest contributors to climate change. Forty percent of the food in our kitchens is thrown into the trash. If food waste were a country, it would be the third-largest emitter of greenhouse gases after the United States and China. Produce thrown in the garbage emits more than 3 times as much methane as factory-farmed livestock. Microplastics that come from waste thrown into the ocean end up in our fish, seafood, and even things like tea, salt, beer, bottled and tap water, and more. Does this mean we should panic? No. It means we need to live as sustainably as possible, and part of that includes how we grow, consume, and discard food and food-related products. Remember, whatever diet we choose (vegan, vegetarian, Paleo, and everything in between), we can move toward a regenerative and protective way of eating—for ourselves and the planet.

ARE PLANT-BASED MEATS THE ANSWER TO CLIMATE CHANGE?

The current buzz about plant-based meats is a distraction. The benefits are dubious at best and the risks unclear. Yes, we should all be eating more plant-rich foods — whole foods, not industrial science projects with GMO ingredients, novel proteins, and a dose of weed killer, also known as glyphosate (a carcinogenic microbiome destroyer), thrown in for good measure. Yes, a soy burger is far better than a feedlot burger, but it turns out that eating a regeneratively raised beef burger removes 3.5 kg of CO_2 from the atmosphere while the Impossible Burger (GMO soy) adds 3.5 kg of CO_2.[23] An independent life cycle analysis by the sustainability experts at Quantis found you would have to eat one regeneratively raised beef burger to offset the carbon emissions of one GMO soy Impossible Burger. Instead of eating Frankenmeats, make your own bean or lentil burger. Have a tempeh sandwich! Stick to real, whole foods, not Frankenfoods.

We explore an optimal vegan diet in Principle 14. If you're a meat eater, choose grass-fed regeneratively raised meat whenever you can, and the next best is grass-finished. As demand increases, so will supply, and prices will drop. If you eat fish, choose wild and sustainably harvested fish, and fish that are not endangered. Choosing meat, poultry, and fish that are raised sustainably, using regenerative practices, not only contributes to the reversal of global warming but also creates better, more nutrient-dense food for you.

PRINCIPLE 9 TAKEAWAYS

1. **Shop local and organic.** Join a community-supported agriculture (CSA) program in your area for local organic produce. Go to Local Harvest (localharvest.org) to find one in your area. Shop at farmers' markets too. They support local food systems.

2. **Look for the new regenerative organic certified (ROC) label.** ROC involves three areas: soil health, animal welfare, and social fairness.

3. **End food waste.** Start a compost pile. Buy only what you need. Eat your leftovers and learn to make WIIF meals (whatever is in the fridge). I'm surprised to hear people say they have nothing to make, and when I look in their pantries and refrigerators, I see a world of possibilities. Try using something like FreshPaper to keep your vegetables and fruits fresher for longer. Check out Imperfect Produce or Misfits to buy fresh but not quite perfect produce at a discount price — produce that's typically tossed into landfills. See the Resources section on page 245 for more information.

4. **Limit your use of plastics.** All of the plastics we throw out are contributing to environmental pollution. Ninety-one percent of plastic is not recycled,[24] even much of what's put in recycling bins. Instead, use glass containers. Take reusable coffee cups to your favorite coffee shop. Pack utensils with you. It might seem frivolous, but it's important.

5. **Eat real, whole foods.** Avoiding packaged, ultra-processed food makes you a climate activist!

Treat Sugar Like a Recreational Drug

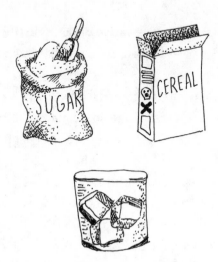

We can all admit that sugar tastes yummy, but it is deadly when overconsumed. The dose makes the poison. A sweet treat occasionally is harmless for most of us, but America is a nation of sugar addicts consuming 152 pounds per person each year. That's an average of almost half a pound of bad stuff per day, and that doesn't include flour (another 133 pounds a year per person), which is even worse than sugar for your body.

THE SCIENCE OF SUGAR ADDICTION

Why is sugar so detrimental? First, we have hundreds of genes protecting us from starvation but few protecting us from abundance or overconsumption. If our ancestors were lucky, they raided a beehive for honey or found a patch of berries that lasted a few weeks at the end of summer. Now we live in a sea of sugar, which causes our biology, especially our hormones, brain chemistry, and immune system, to go haywire, increasing cravings and fat storage (in our belly and around our organs), slowing our metabolism, and fueling our epidemic of obesity, heart disease, diabetes, cancer, and dementia. It all comes down to insulin resistance. One in 2 Americans, including 1 in 4 teenagers, has prediabetes or type 2 diabetes. It used to be called adult-onset diabetes. Not anymore. Why is 75 percent of America (and increasingly the world) overweight? It's sugar and starch, not fat, that is killing us all.

Despite knowing that sugar will wreck our health, we keep eating it. Why? It's biologically addictive. Our bodies are programmed to crave and seek out sugar and store it as fat for the hard winter ahead. But unlike in *Game of Thrones,* winter never comes. The summer of sugar never fades. Imagine crack on every street corner for pennies a dose. Sugar addiction is a biological disorder, driven by hormones and neurotransmitters that fuel cravings and affect the same brain pleasure centers as heroin or cocaine. I imagine you have never binged on a bag of avocados. Cookies always seem to have a habit of disappearing.

Unless you have ever done a sugar detox, you will not likely be able to self-regulate and enjoy a sweet treat once in a while. Taking a break and resetting your hormones, brain, and immune system helps to reset your relationship with sugar. Of course I eat sugar. The key is to make yourself metabolically resilient. How? Start with the Pegan Diet, exercise, and taking active steps to manage your stress levels. Yes, stress can make your blood sugar spike too!

Once or twice a year, I do a sugar detox to reset my body. It's called the *10-Day Reset*. It's not a quick fix. It's not a deprivation diet. It's a system that works using real, whole foods, the right nutrients, and the right habits to reset your system and support healthy blood sugar. We'll talk more about this in Principle 13. If you are overweight, are prediabetic, or have type 2 diabetes, a longer-term reset is needed to repair your metabolism. For some, even a little sugar can trigger a negative spiral. Genetic variations in sweet taste, dopamine pleasure, and other key factors predispose some to cravings, addiction, and overeating.

A healthy relationship with sugar is when you don't crave it or need it every day. Think of sugar as a recreational drug or treat. I love a glass of wine or a little tequila now and then, but I don't have it every day, or for breakfast, lunch, and dinner. Similarly, sugar is a once-in-a-while food, not for every day, or every meal. However, there are a few categories of sugar that I recommend you cut out completely.

DO NOT CONSUME HIGH-FRUCTOSE CORN SYRUP

High-fructose corn syrup (HFCS) is an industrial food product that is far from natural. It's extracted from corn stalks through a chemical enzymatic process. Regular sugar is made of equal parts glucose and fructose. High-fructose corn syrup contains 55 percent fructose and 45 percent glucose (and some HFCS has 75 percent fructose), making it sweeter and more addictive. The reason this stuff is so ubiquitous in processed food is because it's cheap to make (thanks to subsidies). Cheaper and sweeter means more profit and more customers. Since high-fructose corn syrup hit the market, we've seen increased rates of obesity, fatty liver disease, diabetes, and chronic illnesses, especially in children who drink soda. In fact, the number one cause of fatty liver disease in children is drinking soda, because of high-fructose corn syrup. Constant consumption of this poison punches holes in your intestine, leading to leaky gut and driving inflammation. HFCS should be avoided at all costs, not only because of its fructose content, but also because it is almost always found in poor-quality, highly processed food-like substances.

NOT SO FAST WITH THE FAKE SUGAR OR SUGAR SUBSTITUTES

Artificial sweeteners are just as bad as and maybe even worse than regular sugar.[25] How could that be? There are no calories, but remember, food is information, not just calories. Hyper-sweet designer molecules (1,000 times as sweet as regular sugar) adversely impact your brain, hormones, and even microbiome. We have bought into the food industry's manufactured slick halo of zero-calorie foods with Splenda, NutraSweet, Equal, Sweet'N Low, and sugar alcohols. Artificial sweeteners rewire your brain, fuel obesity and belly fat, and are highly addictive. I would rather everyone take a little bit of sugar or honey in their coffee or tea than use packets of artificial sweeteners daily.

Avoid sugar alcohols like erythritol, sorbitol, maltitol, and mannitol. These are not digested and can ferment in your gut, causing diarrhea, bloating, and gas. If you have gut dysbiosis or any digestive issues like irritable bowel syndrome, it is especially important to stay away from sugar alcohols.

Sugar substitutes such as whole plant stevia and monk fruit are better choices. They're great for baking, but use them sparingly. A little bit of honey, high-quality maple syrup, or coconut sugar is fine in small doses like a teaspoon here or there. It's typically not the amount of sugar we add to our coffee or food that's the problem (unless we are baking with cups of sugar); it's the hidden sugar in every processed food from salad dressing to bread that causes trouble. Sugar in cookies I get. But in tomato sauce? There's more sugar in a serving of tomato sauce than in two Oreo cookies.

This table highlights which sugar is safe to consume occasionally and which types should be avoided altogether.

Enjoy in Limited Quantities	Remove or Reduce
Monk fruit	Artificial sweeteners (Splenda, NutraSweet, Equal, Sweet'N Low, etc.)
Organic whole-leaf stevia (not Pure Via or Truvia — made by Pepsi and Coke)	Sugar alcohols
Date sugar	High-fructose corn syrup
Honey	Refined white sugar
Maple syrup	Brown sugar
Coconut sugar	
Molasses	
Fresh fruit juice (4 ounces max, not every day, and not on an empty stomach)	

PRINCIPLE 10 TAKEAWAYS

1. **Remember, sugar is a recreational drug.** It is not a necessary food group. If you want to enjoy safe forms of sugar, that's fine. A little bit of honey in your tea or coffee is fine. Some dessert once or twice a week is totally fine too. I personally enjoy a little bit of dark chocolate daily, but I don't go overboard, and I don't eat sugar for breakfast, lunch, and dinner. Eat sugar at the end of whole food, nutrient-dense meals (the Pegan Diet) to blunt its harmful effects. However, if you know a little sugar will become a slippery slope for overeating, or will trigger addictive behavior, stay away. It may take time to make you metabolically resilient. Try sweetening meals with whole fruit.

2. **Reset your relationship with sugar.** Try giving it up for 10 days and notice how you feel. If you need help, check out the 10-Day Reset. You can find more information about this in Principle 13.

3. **Throw out your Splenda, NutraSweet, and Equal.** If you have to ask whether X is safe (other than what's noted above), the answer is no.

4. **Do not consume high-fructose corn syrup, ever.** Kids do not need soda or diet soda. If they love soda, transition them to sparkling water, very slightly fruit juice–sweetened sparkling drinks such as Spindrift, or healthier soda alternatives like Zevia, which uses stevia as the sweetener.

Don't Rely on Coffee and Alcohol

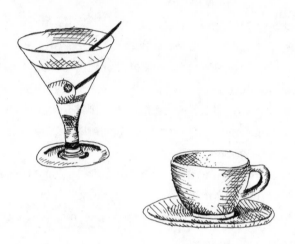

If you have to rely on coffee to wake up in the morning and a glass of wine to wind down at night, it's time to reset. That's not to say you shouldn't enjoy these beverages. I enjoy coffee and a glass of wine or a cocktail now and then, but I don't depend on them. Dependence on coffee and alcohol can interfere with your hormones, sleep, mood, and more. There's only one beverage you need to be healthy, and it's called water.

Our bodies are mostly made up of water; if we don't replenish often, our health suffers. If you're not a huge fan of plain water, you can try adding a little lemon or lime or cucumber to a big pitcher of water to encourage hydration throughout the day. Make iced herbal teas. Sparkling water is Pegan approved, but nothing replaces good old-fashioned plain still water. If I'm working out or super active, I like to add electrolytes to my water. Electrolytes are minerals that help with nerve and muscle function as well as hydration, balancing pH, rebuilding tissue, and removing waste. Adding them to your water can help with adequate hydration and replenishing lost minerals after sweating or working out. They come in drops or powders, and you can find them at Whole Foods, your local health food store, or online. You might notice that hydration alone is enough to make you feel a little more energized. Instead of waking up in the morning and reaching for coffee, drink a glass of filtered water and try adding some electrolytes too.

COFFEE

Coffee is actually the greatest source of antioxidants in the American diet—goes to show how few antioxidants we consume! That's not to say coffee doesn't have some benefits. Studies show that it may reduce the risk of heart disease, dementia, and Parkinson's disease.[26] Here's the challenge: Coffee does not work for everyone. It can increase insulin production in individuals who have type 2 diabetes. It can also create a cascade of hormonal damage by raising cortisol and other stress hormones.

If you drink coffee and feel wired and tired, or experience energy challenges, insomnia, or heart palpitations, you might want to rethink your morning cup of joe. It's wise for everyone to go on a coffee break at least a few times a year. Many of us are far too dependent on caffeine to get our day started. You should be able to have a productive day without coffee. If you want to wean yourself off coffee, try switching to one cup, then half a cup, then green tea. Tea is a super beverage that contains potent phenolic compounds that fight cancer and protect our cardiovascular system. Green tea is in a class by itself, rich in catechins, some of the most powerful disease-fighting phytonutrients found in the plant kingdom. Try a cup or two a day. If you can't live without coffee, avoid all dairy creamers, fake creamers, and sugar-laden Frappuccinos and mochawhatafrappalattes.

ALCOHOL

The simple truth is that alcohol is likely not "good" for anyone. All of the benefits of red wine, such as resveratrol, can be found in other foods and supplements. Consuming more than two alcoholic beverages a day can increase your risk of premature death. Women are even more impacted by the deleterious effects of alcohol than men. There are studies linking alcohol consumption to breast cancer. It depletes nutrients and harms your gut, your liver, and your brain. I've been wearing an Oura ring, which tracks my sleep every night. If I drink alcohol, I notice that it takes me twice as long to fall asleep, my heart rate stays elevated into the night, and I don't feel great the next day. While it might make you feel more relaxed to have a glass of wine at night, I think you'd be surprised to see what alcohol does to your body while you're sleeping. Sleep is when we detoxify and repair; we don't need to make it harder by adding alcohol, a toxin, to the mix.

I treat alcohol like I treat sugar: An occasional glass is fine, but daily can be problematic. Stick to one serving three or four times a week at most. A serving is 1 ounce of hard liquor, 5 ounces of wine, or 10 ounces of beer. If you don't feel great drinking alcohol, skip it altogether. There is no shame in telling people that you don't drink. If someone peer pressures you, be firm about saying no, and tell them that you've been feeling really good while not drinking. No one can argue with that.

A NOTE ABOUT JUICES, SMOOTHIES, AND NUT MILKS

We've seen a massive bump in prepackaged juices and smoothies over the last few years, which is a good sign. It means more people are looking for healthier options. But don't let these prepackaged imposters fool you. Most juices available on the market contain a ton of sugar. A friend was drinking a green smoothie from a popular brand, and I asked to see the label. There were 14 grams of sugar per serving, and the bottle had two servings! That's just a little less than a can of soda. The same goes for green juices containing loads of apple and tropical fruits. If you want green juice, stick with the ones that are just greens and a little bit of lemon and ginger. If you want a smoothie, best to make it yourself or purchase it from a company that uses only whole real ingredients. Make sure it doesn't contain isolated soy protein, which may be harmful, unlike whole traditional soy products such as tempeh, tofu, or miso. I like to get fresh smoothies from Whole Foods and other health food stores, and I ask them to make them with avocado, greens, berries, protein powder, and almond milk. You don't need bananas, dates, and agave in your smoothie; this is just extra sugar. When it comes to nut milk, seek out the brands with the fewest ingredients, or make your own.

PRINCIPLE 11 TAKEAWAYS

1. **Prioritize plain filtered water above all other beverages.** Add electrolytes if you're working out vigorously or after something like hot yoga. You can get a liquid or powdered version to add to your water. I list my favorite brands in the Resources section on page 245.
2. **Caffeinated tea and coffee are okay if you don't get the jitters or adverse reactions.** Green tea has the most benefits.
3. **Avoid all sugar-sweetened and artificially sweetened beverages.** Full stop.
4. **Limit alcohol to one glass of wine or one cocktail three to four times a week.** I recommend skipping beer since it typically contains gluten and a big load of carbohydrates (hence the familiar "beer belly").

Leverage Personalized Nutrition for Optimal Health

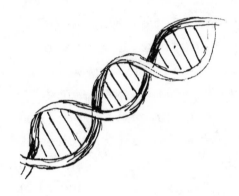

Imagine a future (a not too distant one) when you collect a cheek swab, a few drops of blood, and a little poop, which are analyzed. Then you're given a map of the unique genetic, biochemical, metabolic, and even microbial creature that is you. Driven through massive databases, interpreted by artificial intelligence, complemented by real-time wearables that measure your vital signs, blood sugar, and more, this information will herald a new era of personalized and precision nutrition. What foods will optimize your metabolism? What foods turn on your healing genes and turn off your disease-causing genes? What is your unique need for nutrients? How do you feed your particular microbiome? Which of the tens of thousands of phytochemicals in food will benefit you the most?

That day will come soon enough, but today, there's a lot you can do to discover the right diet and nutrient intake for you. It is what I have been doing for 30 years with my patients. Today's tools are good, and while better ones are coming fast, blood tests, hormone levels, nutrient levels, genetic tests, microbiome analysis, and food sensitivity testing can get you pretty close to precision nutrition.

If eating were all about calories, life would be fairly simple. But food is not just calories or energy; food is information, instructions that upgrade or downgrade your biology with every bite. Think of it like code that programs your software. Your hardware is your genes. Your software is how those genes are turned on or off. Food regulates not only your genes but also your hormones, like insulin, testosterone, estrogen, and thyroid. It alters your brain chemistry, producing happy chemicals, and it can even trigger addictive patterns. You feed the 100 trillion bacteria living inside you with every bite and grow good bugs or bad. Food can create or stop inflammation, enhance or hurt your immune system. It provides the raw materials for your muscles, bones, brain, and every other part of your body.

So how can you personalize your diet (and nutritional needs)? There are six ways I help my patients personalize their diet.

1. **Personal history and family history.** If you struggle with belly fat or resistance to weight loss, or have a family history of obesity, diabetes, dementia, heart disease, autoimmune diseases, or allergies, for example, I know where the pitfalls are. You may be

more likely to be carbohydrate intolerant, or need to avoid saturated fats, or be at risk for gluten sensitivity.

2. **Hormonal and metabolic testing.** Measuring lipids, insulin, and blood sugar helps guide my recommendations. Are you more likely to pile on the pounds on a carbohydrate-rich diet, or should you completely avoid saturated fat?

3. **Nutritional testing.** Most physicians don't measure nutrient levels. Since 90 percent of Americans are deficient in one or more nutrients at the minimum level to prevent deficiency diseases, testing is a good idea. The most common deficiencies are omega-3 fats, vitamin D, magnesium, folate, B_{12}, zinc, and iron. Easy to fix yet often missed. Nutrients regulate every single chemical reaction in your body. How many is that? Thirty-seven billion billion reactions—every second! When you have less than optimal levels of these nutrients, your metabolic machinery slows down. The result—feeling crappy, or worse, chronic disease.

4. **Food allergy and sensitivity testing.** While there is a lot of controversy about allergy and food sensitivity testing, it can be very useful when interpreted properly. The most common foods that cause problems are gluten and dairy. Others include eggs, corn, soy, grains, beans, and sometimes nightshades (tomatoes, peppers, potatoes, eggplant) and nuts. Lots of sensitivities often indicate a leaky gut, with all these proteins leaking into the bloodstream, causing a reaction. Fixing the gut fixes the sensitivities.

5. **Stool testing.** It sounds fun, I know, but stool testing can tell you a lot about the state of your gut health. The microbiome plays a significant role in your health and metabolism. Some findings from testing are easy to support, such as low levels of short-chain fatty acids, beneficial fuel for the gut, which can be increased by consuming pre- and probiotic foods. Other findings may show low levels of immune-regulatory bugs, which feed on cranberry, pomegranate, and green tea.

6. **Genetic testing.** While we have much to learn, we know there are many genes that regulate your metabolism and how you handle fats and carbohydrates, and that are linked to appetite, taste preferences, predisposition to food addiction, and how food and nutrients optimize your gene expression. You may be like me and be a poor detoxifier and require regular doses of cruciferous veggies such as kale and broccoli. Or you may have genes that predispose you to inflammation and could benefit from turmeric and fish oil. Or you may have genes that require you to take higher doses of vitamin D, folate, or vitamin B_{12}. Genes are not destiny, but they are important. Genetics loads the gun, but your environment (diet, lifestyle, exposures, etc.) pulls the trigger.

Some of these tests are not common in a conventional medicine practice. I know that not everyone has access to a functional medicine practitioner, but there are ways to personalize your diet at home and work with your doctor to get the tests you need to modify your diet. The Pegan Diet Principles are the foundation for everyone. If you're still experiencing symptoms and want to dial in your personal needs, start with these steps.

START WITH THE ELIMINATION DIET

Certain foods cause an array of symptoms, or what I call FLC (feel like crap) syndrome—bloating, eczema, allergies, fatigue, brain fog, headaches, autoimmune disease, and systemic inflammation. They can include gluten, wheat, dairy, soy, grains, beans, nightshades, eggs, sugar, and caffeinated beverages. These are not problematic for everyone, but the key is to identify if they are a trigger for you. Eliminate these foods for 21 days. On day 22, start by introducing one food at a time. For example, if you suspect that gluten is an issue, try eating a piece of bread or some pasta on days 22 and 23 while sticking with the elimination diet. Wait 24 hours and notice how you feel. This is a lengthy process. However, it is the gold standard to personalize diet. If you know that other foods bother you, then stop those too. If you're unsure where to start, remove gluten, wheat, dairy, and sugar first.

WORK WITH YOUR DOCTOR TO GET WHAT YOU NEED

One of the best ways to determine whether or not your diet is working for you is to assess your metabolic health. I recommend asking your doctor about an NMR lipid test, fasting insulin and glucose, and your six-week average blood sugar or hemoglobin A1c. If your blood sugar or insulin comes back high, this is an opportunity to reevaluate your diet. Often, high insulin and blood sugar are the results of too many starches and sugars, too much stress, and not enough movement. If your lipids appear abnormal and you're on a high-fat diet, this is a clue that saturated fats or a large amount of fat doesn't work for your body. You can instead ease up on fats and eat more whole food carbohydrates from plant foods, such as veggies, fruit, beans, whole grains, nuts, and seeds. Tests don't lie, and they are an easy way to get feedback about your diet.

Nutrient levels are also key, yet most physicians don't measure them. Since 90 percent of Americans are deficient in one or more nutrients at the minimum level to prevent deficiency diseases like scurvy, testing is a good idea. Ask your doctor to measure your omega-3 levels, vitamin D, plasma zinc, red blood cell magnesium, iron (ferritin), and homocysteine and methylmalonic acid, which are functional tests for assessing folate and B_{12} deficiencies.

Another way to understand if your diet is working for you is to check for delayed food sensitivities and allergies. The elimination diet is a perfect first step, but if you're not having luck identifying where your symptoms are coming from, try a food sensitivity test. If you have a chronic or inflammatory disease, you should check gluten antibodies. IgG and sometimes IgA blood tests measure antibodies to common food antigens. These antibodies can result from leaky gut, which allows food proteins to "leak" into your bloodstream, triggering an immune reaction. A healing gut protocol, explained in Principle 15, can reduce sensitivities and help expand your diet.

EXPLORE GENETIC TESTING

If you've done a test like 23andMe, I recommend running your results through a program that can give you very specific information on nutritional changes that will impact you. You can upload your data to Genetic Genie (geneticgenie .org).

Knowing your unique needs can help you design a way of eating, a personalized supplement regimen, and an exercise plan to help you thrive. If your genes increase your risk for insulin resistance or inflammation, don't panic. By understanding your risks, you can modify how those genes are expressed by controlling the *exposome*—the sum total of everything that washes over your genes: your diet, lifestyle, stress, sleep, exercise, microbes, allergens, toxins, and so on. It turns out the exposome, not your genes, determines 90 percent of all chronic disease.

PRINCIPLE 12 TAKEAWAYS

1. **The Pegan Diet Principles are the foundation for everyone.** Eat whole, nutrient-dense food, low-glycemic food, plant-rich food, good fats, and high-quality protein. Often just this alone will improve your health dramatically. If you still feel off and want to take it further, follow the next steps.

2. **Do an elimination diet for 21 days.** If you're just getting started on your health journey, remove wheat, gluten, dairy, and sugar. If you've already taken these out of your diet, try removing soy, grains, beans, nightshades, eggs, and caffeinated beverages. Reintroduce each food one at a time to see if any symptoms come up. If they do, you might need to temporarily

remove that food from your diet. If you're still feeling lost after the elimination diet, consider getting a food sensitivity test.

3. **Get the right tests.** Ask your doctor to run an NMR lipid test, fasting insulin and glucose, and hemoglobin A1c. Also ask your doctor to run nutrient testing to see if you're deficient in critical vitamins, minerals, and nutrients.

4. **Try genetic testing.** There are so many great resources out there like 23andMe and Genetic Genie to help you identify which diet is best for you. Sometimes to fit into your jeans, you have to fit into your genes.

5. **Find a functional medicine doctor.** When you feel like you've tried everything and are not seeing results, it might be time to work with a functional medicine practitioner. You can visit ifm.org to find a doctor in your area. My clinic is also taking virtual appointments. Visit ultrawellnesscenter.com for more information.

Cleanse, Detox, and Reset Wisely

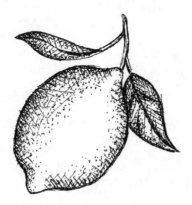

While most people have not experienced the healing power of food, there is no more powerful drug on the planet. It is the main medicine I use to treat my patients, and it works better than almost any other drug for most of our common chronic conditions, like diabetes, dementia, depression, autoimmune disease, and digestive disorders. While working with a trained functional medicine practitioner can help guide your journey, there is a lot you can do on your own. Food can heal you.

For most of us, the best place to start is a simple reset. I do one as each season changes or if I have been traveling and feel sluggish or run-down. Over the years, I've tried many detoxes and juice cleanses, and while they can be valuable, they are not sustainable. The best reset is not a quick fix. It is something that sets you up for long-term success. It helps you make the very real connection between what you eat and how you feel.

This is why I created the 10-Day Reset—a program based on what has worked for most of my patients over 30 years of practicing functional medicine. It is designed to reboot your biology, reduce cravings, reduce inflammation, optimize your gut health, and support healthy blood sugar. It's a whole food–based, low-glycemic, anti-inflammatory, gut-healing, detoxifying, phytochemical-rich diet. Whether you struggle with weight loss challenges, sugar addiction, prediabetes, metabolic syndrome, or FLC (feel like crap) syndrome, the 10-Day Reset works. We thrive when we feed our bodies the right information, but we all get off track once in a while. Don't listen to me. Listen to your body. The results from a simple reset don't take weeks or months. The changes start within a few days. You will be able to choose how you feel, rather than be tossed around in a fog of symptoms and confusion about how your diet affects your well-being.

The reset relies on a combination of foods and habits that are critical for supporting detoxification and rebooting your body—what you eat, when you eat, and when you sleep. Let's break each of these down.

WHAT YOU EAT

Food is foundational when it comes to supporting our healing journey. The first step of the reset is to *take out* potentially harmful foods and *add in* an abundance of real, whole foods. This is similar to the elimination diet I discussed in Principle 12. The key here is to focus on nutrient-dense foods while removing foods that fuel inflammation and sugar addiction.

	Eat This	Don't Eat That
Meats, poultry, and eggs	Pasture-raised chicken, turkey, duck, pheasant, Cornish game hen; pasture-raised and organic eggs; grass-fed, pasture-raised lamb, beef, bison, venison, ostrich, deer, elk	Conventionally raised chicken, duck, eggs, turkey; all processed meats and deli meats; conventionally raised bacon, beef, hot dogs, lamb, pork, sausage, salami
Fish and seafood	Anchovies, clams, cod, crab, flounder/sole, herring, small halibut, mussels, wild salmon (canned or fresh), sardines, sable, shrimp, scallops, trout	Larger fish like halibut, Chilean sea bass, tuna, swordfish; farm-raised fish
Nuts and seeds	Nuts: almonds, Brazil nuts, cashews, hazelnuts, macadamias, pecans, pine nuts, pistachios, walnuts, raw cacao	Nuts with sugar or chocolate, nut butters that contain hydrogenated oils or sugar, peanuts/peanut butter
	Seeds: chia, flax, hemp, pumpkin, sesame, sunflower	
	Nut/seed butters and flours: unsweetened almond, cashew, pecan, macadamia, walnut, coconut	
Oils	Grass-fed ghee; humanely raised tallow, lard, duck fat, chicken fat; organic avocado oil; organic virgin coconut oil; almond oil; flax oil; hemp oil; macadamia oil; organic extra virgin olive oil (low- or medium-heat cooking); sesame seed oil; tahini; walnut oil	Canola oil, partially or fully hydrogenated oils, margarine, peanut oil, soybean oil, sunflower oil, safflower oil, trans fats, vegetable oil, vegetable shortening

Vegetables	Non-starchy: organic artichokes, asparagus, avocado, bean sprouts, broccoli, Brussels sprouts, cabbage, cauliflower, celery, cucumber, eggplant, garlic, ginger root, hearts of palm, kohlrabi, leafy greens, mushrooms, onions, peppers, radicchio, radish, rutabaga, seaweed, shallots, summer squash, tomatoes, turnips, zucchini (unlimited)	
	Starchy: yam, sweet potatoes, winter squash, pumpkin (limited to ½ cup per day)	Corn, white potatoes
Dairy	Grass-fed ghee	All dairy other than grass-fed ghee
Beans	Green beans, green peas, gluten-free soy sauce, lentils, miso, natto, non-GMO soy, tempeh, chickpeas, black beans, snap peas, snow peas	GMO soy, soymilk, soybean oil, peanuts/peanut butter, lima beans, baked beans. Avoid all beans if you have an autoimmune condition, prediabetes or diabetes, or a leaky gut.
Grains	Quinoa (limited to ½ cup per day)	Wheat, barley, rye, rice, amaranth, millet, teff, spelt, kamut, oats, semolina couscous, and all sources of gluten
Fruits	Organic blackberries, blueberries, cranberries, kiwi, lemons, limes, raspberries (limited to ½ cup per day)	High-glycemic fruits: bananas, dried fruit, fruit juice, grapes, mangoes, pineapples, apples, cherries, grapes, nectarines, peaches, pears, strawberries
Sugars and sweeteners		All sugars, sweeteners, and artificial sweeteners
Beverages	Purified water, herbal tea, seltzer, mineral water	Alcohol, coffee, soda, sugary beverages

WHEN YOU EAT

Time-restricted eating has gained popularity over recent years, and for good reason. It has been shown to trigger powerful repair and healing mechanisms in the body—organ- and belly-fat loss, increased lean muscle mass, reduced inflammation and oxidative stress, repair and regeneration of mitochondria (our cells' energy factories), improved cognitive function, enhanced autophagy (how your cells clean up waste), and disease prevention.

Time-restricted eating means eating within a specific time window—12, 10, or 8 hours—and not eating the other 12, 14, or 16 hours of the day. That's why the first meal of the day is called breakfast: We break the fast. If you eat dinner at 6 p.m. and breakfast at 8 a.m., that's a 14-hour fast. Snacking and late-night eating interfere with your body's ability to rest, repair, and regenerate. Time-restricted eating doesn't restrict calories; it limits your feeding window to optimize repair. For example, you might consume all of your meals between 7 a.m. and 3 p.m., or 7 a.m. and 5 p.m. It works no matter what you eat, but it works far better when you combine it with the 10-Day Reset.

Really narrow windows of time, like eating only within an 8-hour window, are not always the best choice if you're already thin, chronically fatigued, or pregnant, or have an eating disorder. But there is a form of fasting that most of us can and should do every day—the 12-hour window: 12 hours between your last meal of the day and your first meal of the next day. The 12-hour window allows your body to have a natural period of rest and detoxification. While you follow the 10-Day Reset, apply the 12-hour window and consider expanding to 14 or even 16 hours depending on how you feel.

WHEN YOU SLEEP

Your circadian rhythm regulates your sleep-wake cycle and is largely controlled by light exposure, exercise, food, and stress—all things we can influence with lifestyle changes. I believe that sleep is the most underrated pillar of wellness. It's crucial for increasing longevity, energy, focus, and brain health, reducing the risk of Alzheimer's and dementia, clearing toxins, storing memories, healing vital organs, and improving learning. Think about what happens when you don't get quality sleep or have a restless night. I don't know about you, but I feel completely useless the next day. Dialing in your sleep routine is so essential to restoration and detoxification that I made it an essential part of my 10-Day Reset. And a few simple habits can transform your sleep. During the 10-Day Reset, follow these simple rules.

1. Set a bedtime and try to stick to it. I know that I want to start to wind down around 9 and to be in bed by 10 every day.
2. Put your phone on airplane mode, shut off the TV, and put away all devices 45 minutes before bed.
3. Use the remaining time to focus on active relaxation. This can include reading, journaling, meditation, or meaningful conversation with loved ones. I like to have a hot bath around 8:30 p.m. Then I read for a little while and write in my gratitude journal.

4. Get exposure to sunlight in the morning. Believe it or not, one of the best ways to reset your circadian rhythm is to expose yourself to about 15 minutes of sunlight in the morning. Instead of looking at your phone first thing, try a meditation or walk outside. Try to get outside a few times a day. At night, close to bedtime, keep lighting dim. Low lighting sends a signal to your body that it's time to sleep. Try blue light–blocking glasses after the sun goes down.

There's no shortage of cleanses and detoxes out there designed to help you lose weight and feel better quickly. But the most powerful, simplest, and most delicious reset is available to anyone, anywhere, anytime by eating real, whole, fresh food and incorporating a few simple habits. The root cause of most modern illness is a result of hyper-processed, addictive food that hijacks our taste buds, brain chemistry, and metabolism. The 10-Day Reset works because it removes all of these food–like substances and addictive foods for just 10 days, so the body can reboot and reset. Think of it as turning your body back to its original factory settings.

WHAT ABOUT SUPPLEMENTS?

For years doctors recommended that you get all your vitamins and minerals from food. As the role of nutrients in preventing and treating chronic disease has become better understood, 72 percent of physicians now recommend nutritional supplements for their patients, and 79 percent take supplements themselves.[27] Cardiologists recommend fish oil and CoQ10. Gastroenterologists prescribe gut-healing probiotics. Our modern nutrient-depleted diets, depleted soils, toxic exposures, and increased demands from stressful lifestyles make it harder to get nutrients from what we eat.

I don't guess what my patients need; I test. Most of my patients are deficient in one or more critical nutrients. Nearly 80 percent of Americans are deficient in or have insufficient levels of vitamin D — critical for immunity, bone building, mood, and energy (and preventing and treating COVID-19). National government nutritional studies have found that 92 percent of Americans have at least one vitamin or mineral deficiency. The most common are omega-3 fats, vitamin D, zinc, iron, folate, and magnesium. Each nutrient regulates hundreds of biochemical pathways. Both obese and diabetic patients are often malnourished, and surprisingly, the most obese are often the most nutrient-deficient. Eating nutrient-depleted food makes us seek even more food to find those nutrients. Studies have found that people eat far less when consuming nutrient-dense whole foods than when eating processed foods. In one study, one group on a processed food diet ate 500 more calories a day than another group on a whole foods diet, even though the diets had the same amount of protein, fat, carbohydrates, sugar, sodium, and fiber. They were looking to get more nutrients in food without any, so they kept eating more. It's like looking for love in all the wrong places!

Nutrients are essential for getting the body back into balance. We need supplements to thrive and to bounce back when struggling with chronic illness. But there are tons of shady supplements on the market, so treat your supplements like you treat your food — only the best! I recommend a high-quality multivitamin and mineral supplement, fish oil, vitamin D, magnesium, and probiotics for daily use. The focus of the Pegan

Diet and the 10-Day Reset is food, but supplements are also critical. If you want to know more about what supplements and which brands I recommend for daily use, see the Resources section on page 245. If you want to support your 10-Day Reset with the supplements that I recommend, check out getfarmacy.com.

PRINCIPLE 13 TAKEAWAYS

1. **Follow the "Eat This" approved foods for 10 days.** Remove the "Don't Eat That" foods.
2. **Follow the 12- or 14-hour window.** Eat your last meal at least 2 hours before bed, and give yourself at least 12 or 14 hours between dinner and breakfast.
3. **Set up a sleep schedule.** Commit to a bedtime daily. Turn off electronics at least 45 minutes before bed and spend the time before you sleep on active relaxation, such as taking a hot Epsom salt bath or practicing yoga, deep breathing, or meditation.

Assess the Risks and Benefits of a Vegan Diet

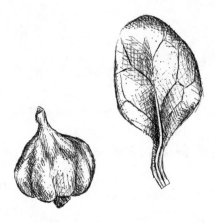

The impact of a vegan diet vs. an omnivore diet is more nuanced than meat is terrible for our health and the planet, and a vegan diet will save us from disease and climate change. In fact, the science is clear: integrating animals into food production is essential for environmental and climate restoration. In Principle 5 I reviewed the science of meat and health. Feedlot meat is bad. Regenerative, grass-fed, or wild meat in the context of a plant- and spice-rich whole foods diet promotes health and is better for the environment and climate than a plant foods–only diet. However, whether it be for ethical, religious, or moral reasons, or simply just preference, there are plenty of individuals who feel better eating a vegan diet. Is it possible to be a vegan on the Pegan Diet? Yes. Is it easy? Not really. I respect the choice to be a vegan or vegetarian. I was vegan for more than ten years. I support my vegan patients who want to optimize their health. In this principle, I'm going to synthesize my biggest concerns about a vegan diet and suggest how you can optimize your animal-free diet with the right steps.

ADDRESS NUTRITIONAL DEFICIENCIES

While a vegan diet can be healthful for many, it is often fraught with challenges and doesn't fulfill the biological needs of humans. By definition, a vegan diet is deficient in certain essential nutrients—omega-3 fats (DHA and EPA), vitamin B_{12}, vitamin D, iodine, iron, and zinc. The protein concentration and quality are lower in plants than in animal products and may not adequately preserve and build muscles as we age.

As a practicing physician, I don't just read the science; I see patients, and it is humbling. Most vegetarians or vegans who switch from a processed food American diet to a whole food plant-based diet do very well initially. But over time they develop vitamin and mineral deficiencies and low levels of essential omega-3 fats (even if they eat flax, hemp, chia, and walnuts, which contain a plant-based source of omega-3 called ALA that is not easily converted to EPA and DHA). They often complain of low energy and low libido. Even if they lose weight, they may develop insulin resistance, lose muscle, and develop prediabetes because of increased carbohydrate and reduced protein intakes. Vegans who eat a junk food diet of chips and soda fare far worse.

I'm committed to making everyone healthy, regardless of their dietary, moral, or ethical beliefs. Lab testing is essential. What are your nutrient levels? Consider getting a full nutritional evaluation from a functional medicine provider. My favorite tests are from Genova Labs (the NutrEval or the ION panel). These tests provide a detailed analysis of vitamins, minerals, fatty acids, antioxidant levels, organic acids, and amino acids and can guide you on supplementation. Make a decision about your diet based on your biology, your numbers, and how you feel.

EAT REAL FOOD, NOT FRANKENFOOD

Now, be honest: Are you a chips-and-soda vegan or a plant-rich vegan? Really take a look at your dietary habits. I find that most young adults who are committed to cruelty-free living fall into the chips-and-soda vegan category. They come to my office complaining of acne, bad PMS, fatigue, digestive problems, or worse. When we review their diet, I find that it's riddled with refined cereal grains, starches, sugars, and refined vegetable oils. Many of my Paleo patients eat more fresh vegetables and fruits than my vegan patients!

Keep a food journal. Bad dietary habits can be insidious—maybe some oatmeal for breakfast, a sandwich for lunch, and then a big bowl of pasta for dinner. If that sounds like your diet, step one is to reset your eating habits. Remember, being Pegan means sticking to real, whole foods; it means eating a plant-rich diet. Commit to taking all Frankenfoods and food-like substances out of your diet. This means all fake meats, hydrogenated products, processed foods with vegetable oils, and vegan pastries and bread with loads of ingredients. After you eliminate the Frankenfoods, add in the good stuff. Replace starch (like bread, pasta, and rice) and sugar with vegan protein like tempeh, tofu, lentils, and low-starch beans (like lupini beans) and nutrient-dense whole grains such as quinoa, black rice, buckwheat, amaranth, and teff. Follow all the principles of the Pegan Diet but without the animal products.

EAT PROTEIN

My friend and Harvard researcher Dr. David Ludwig recently gave a talk in India (which has a high percentage of vegetarians) in which he discussed why type 2 diabetes, metabolic syndrome, and heart disease are on the rise in South Asia. Ancient and traditional diets, while focused on vegetarian foods, did not contain the amount of starch and bad fats that many vegetarians consume in these modern times. Replacing starch with vegetables, good fats, and protein is essential for vegans.

Speaking of protein, you'll have to eat a lot of beans (hello, gas!) to add up to the amount of protein that you would get from a chicken breast (2 cups of beans equals 4 ounces of chicken). Additionally, proteins from plants are incomplete or are low in certain essential amino acids. Combining nuts and seeds, whole grains, and beans gives you a balance of amino acids.

A complete protein contains all nine essential amino acids. But even good plant proteins are low in branched-chain amino acids necessary for muscle synthesis. To ensure consistent protein intake for my vegan patients (especially athletes), I recommend a protein shake. I like pea, pumpkin, and hemp protein. (You can find some of my favorite brands in the Resources section on page 245, or try my Pegan Shake at getfarmacy.com/pegan.) Make sure that your protein powder has a full amino acid profile that includes a total of 2.5 grams of leucine along with the other branched amino acids, isoleucine and valine. Leucine is the most critical branched-chain amino acid for building muscle. It activates pathways necessary for muscle protein synthesis, which is essential as you age.

For optimal health, in addition to good vegan protein powders, you will need vitamin, mineral, and omega-3 supplements. (You can get pre-formed DHA from algae-based supplements.)

Becoming a healthy vegan comes down to a few basics. You always want to start by reducing starch from refined carbs and upping protein and high-quality fats.

PRINCIPLE 14 TAKEAWAYS

1. **Eat a whole foods, plant-based diet** following the Pegan Principles. Regardless of whether you're vegan or not, most of your plate by volume — 75 percent is the goal — should be non-starchy vegetables. Eat green leafy vegetables, peppers, cucumbers, broccoli, cauliflower, bok choy, and other non-starchy veggies.
2. **Stick to whole kernel grains** instead of processed grains. Add ½ to 1 cup of whole grains, like brown rice, wild rice, quinoa, or buckwheat, to your meals.
3. **Manage insulin and hunger by eating good fats.** Eat avocados, nuts, seeds, and extra virgin olive oil.

4. **Eat protein-rich vegan foods.** My favorite vegan proteins include tempeh, tofu, lentils, lupini beans, and black beans.

5. **Add a protein shake.** Try a pea-, pumpkin-, or hemp-based protein powder. Add a BCAA (branched-chain amino acid) supplement to build muscle. Some protein powders already have a full amino acid profile.

6. **Take supplements.** Ideally, take a multivitamin, vitamin D, omega-3 fats, zinc, iodine, vitamin B_{12}, and, especially for menstruating people, iron supplements.

PRINCIPLE 15

Eat for Gut Health

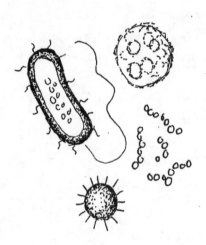

This is the decade, maybe even the century, of the microbiome. Who knew that poop was the key to health, weight loss, and longevity? Hippocrates did when he said, "All disease begins in the gut." While the science of the microbiome is still in its infancy, practitioners of functional medicine have been treating complex chronic diseases by fixing the gut for decades—autoimmune disease, allergies, mood disorders, diabetes, heart disease, cancer, skin problems, headaches, weight issues, hormonal imbalances, and even autism. A fecal transplant, for instance, reduced autistic symptoms by 50 percent in one study, an improvement that lasted long-term.[28]

It turns out the microbiome is likely the most important

regulator of our overall health. There are 100 trillion microbes in you, 10 times the number of your own cells, and 100 times your DNA. We have 20,000 genes. Your microbiome contains 2 to 5 million microbial genes, all making proteins, cell-signaling molecules, messengers of health or disease. Some scientists estimate that a third to half of all the molecules in our blood come from microbial metabolites. They interact with our genes, hormones, immune system, brain chemistry, and every single process in our biology. Our gut microbes also provide us with essential vitamins: vitamin K and biotin.

Sadly, our gut microbiome ain't what it used to be. We eat gut-busting foods, live a gut-busting lifestyle, and take gut-busting drugs. Want to grow toxic weeds in your gut? Feed them a processed diet high in sugar and starch, food additives, and the microbiome-destroying weed killer glyphosate, used on 70 percent of all crops. Our diet is also low in food for the good bugs: prebiotic fibers and polyphenols (all the colorful medicinal compounds in plant foods). We also take too many gut-damaging antibiotics, acid blockers, anti-inflammatories like Advil, hormones, and steroids. Add to that environmental toxins from our food, air, and water, and our inner garden is a sorry place with too many disease-causing bugs and not enough healing bugs.

The bad bugs drive inflammation, which is at the root of almost all chronic diseases and obesity. Sixty percent of your immune system is in your gut, right under a one-cell-thin layer of gut lining. When we treat this lining unkindly, we develop a leaky gut, allowing food proteins, microbes, and microbial toxins to "leak" into our bloodstream, triggering our immune system to start fighting the foreign invaders. Your biology is collateral damage. We call this *dysbiosis* (as opposed to symbiosis), an imbalanced gut microbiome.

Every day we understand more and more about the link between chronic illness and gut dysbiosis. My journey toward understanding is not just theoretical. My own gut taught me much about what goes wrong and how to fix it. Twenty-five years ago, mercury toxicity damaged my intestinal microbiome, resulting in severe irritable bowel syndrome, bloating, and diarrhea. Getting the mercury out and healing my gut fixed it, but I guess I still had more to learn.

Things got really, really bad for my gut a few years ago. It was a perfect storm, a domino effect of insults. It started with a bad root canal treated with the antibiotic clindamycin, which caused a deadly gut infection known as *C. diff* that kills 30,000 people a year. My 24/7 pain, bloody stools, diarrhea, fever, and nausea ultimately led to full-blown ulcerative colitis. Oh, and did I mention I broke my arm at the same time and took anti-inflammatories for the pain, triggering severe gastritis? My digestion was a red-hot inflamed mess from gut to butt. I was down for the count for five months and couldn't work, focus, or even answer an e-mail. I lost 30 pounds. I was so desperate to get better that I took high doses of prednisone, a steroid. It didn't work.

Using the principles of functional medicine, I went deep into innovative strategies to heal and restore my gut health.

The science of the microbiome has advanced so far, so fast, that I created a powerful new method to fix stubborn gut problems. My colitis went away in three weeks. Along with diet and all the other tools of functional medicine, this innovation has been a game changer for my patients with gut problems—everything from mild irritable bowel to full-blown inflammatory bowel disease.

Growing a healthy inner garden helps heal a leaky gut—the root of most inflammatory and chronic diseases. It even helps with obesity. Without changing diets, transplanting bugs from a thin mouse to a fat mouse makes the fat mouse lose weight. Fecal transplants from healthy humans to diabetic ones improve diabetes![29] I know we're not all signing up to do fecal transplants, so here are three steps toward cultivating a healthy inner garden.

1. Weed: Remove gut-busting foods and drugs

Bad bugs love sugar, starch, and processed foods. Ditch the following gut bombs.

- Highly processed or packaged foods
- Refined grains, especially wheat, or all grains or beans if your gut dysbiosis is severe
- Gluten, dairy, and any other foods to which you may be sensitive
- Sugars, especially high-fructose corn syrup, artificial sweeteners, and sugar alcohols
- Refined oils and fats, especially soybean and corn oil

- Antibiotic drugs, except when absolutely necessary
- Steroids
- Anti-inflammatories, including ibuprofen (Advil), naproxen (Aleve), and aspirin
- Acid blockers, like those prescribed for acid reflux
- Chronic stressors (stress causes leaky gut)
- Environmental toxins, especially glyphosate-sprayed products such as wheat and industrial soy and corn products

2. Seed: Add in the good bugs

Include fermented or cultured foods in your diet, such as:

- Naturally fermented sauerkraut
- Pickled vegetables (including pickles)
- Kimchi (fermented vegetables or fruit)
- Kefir (fermented milk, ideally goat or sheep— unsweetened only)
- Miso
- Gluten-free tamari
- Tempeh (fermented soybean cake)
- Tofu (which is sometimes fermented)
- Naturally fermented soy sauce
- Unpasteurized apple cider vinegar
- Coconut yogurt (unsweetened)

3. Feed: Support the growth of healthy bacteria

Include both prebiotic and fiber-rich foods for the gut.

Prebiotic Foods

(If you have small intestinal bacterial overgrowth, these foods might need to be introduced slowly. Too many prebiotic foods all at once can exacerbate symptoms.)

- Apples
- Artichokes
- Asparagus
- Dandelion greens
- Jerusalem artichokes
- Jicama root
- Onions, garlic, and leeks
- Plantains and underripe bananas
- Polyphenol-rich foods like cranberry, pomegranate, and green tea
- Seaweed

Fiber-Rich Foods

- Avocados
- Beans
- Berries
- Broccoli
- Brussels sprouts
- Cabbage
- Celery
- Cucumber
- Figs
- Kale
- Lentils
- Nuts and seeds, especially sprouted

- Olives and olive oil
- Pumpkin
- Spinach
- Strawberries

For severe cases of gut dysbiosis, like mine, I recommend a super shake designed to quickly heal a dysfunctional gut. It cured my colitis in weeks. Synthesizing my 30 years of experience with the latest science on the microbiome, I designed a therapeutic cocktail to heal the gut and grow some very important beneficial bacteria, especially *Akkermansia muciniphila. Akkermansia* supports the protective mucus layer that prevents a leaky gut. Low levels of this critical bacteria have been linked to autoimmune disease, obesity, diabetes, heart disease, and even cancer. I had no *Akkermansia* growing in my gut. You can't take it as a probiotic (yet), and while fiber helps, it turns out *Akkermansia* thrives on colorful polyphenols found in cranberry, pomegranate, and green tea.

The foundation of my inner garden gut shake is polyphenols. They feed the good bugs and inhibit the growth of bad bacteria. I have since prescribed hundreds of patients this shake. It is my secret weapon when other things fail to treat chronic disease. But it can be used by anyone who wants to optimize their gut.

Here's the homemade version. If you want a premade version, visit getfarmacy.com.

Dr. Mark Hyman's Gut-Healing Shake

1 scoop ImmunoG PRP by NuMedica or SBI Protect (dairy-free) by
  Orthomolecular Products (bovine immunoglobulins aka
  colostrum)
1 scoop acacia fiber (a prebiotic)
1 tablespoon pomegranate concentrate (I use Lakewood organic)
1 tablespoon cranberry concentrate (I use Lakewood organic)
1 teaspoon matcha green tea powder (I use Navitas)
1 stick ProbioMax 350 DF by Xymogen (or your favorite high-potency
  probiotic)
1 scoop collagen powder

Blend or mix everything with a cup of water and drink.

Functional medicine practitioners are gut experts. Working
on gut restoration with a functional medicine practitioner
can be a game changer for those with resistant or more
challenging symptoms. You may have bacterial or fungal
overgrowth, or a parasite, or a load of hidden mercury. You
may need a little extra support.

A functional medicine practitioner can investigate your
gut health using stool tests, breath tests for overgrowth of
bad bugs, food sensitivity testing, and customized diets and
healing protocols. Learn more at ultrawellnesscenter.com
to work with my team virtually.

PRINCIPLE 15 TAKEAWAYS

1. **Weed.** Follow the Pegan Diet, and remove all sugars, artificial
   sweeteners, starchy foods, gluten and wheat, and processed

foods. You may need a functional medicine practitioner if you have bad bacterial or yeast overgrowth or parasites.

2. **Seed.** Eat probiotic-rich foods like tempeh, sauerkraut, miso, and kimchi. Or take a daily probiotic.

3. **Feed.** Eat prebiotic- and fiber-rich foods such as garlic, onions, avocado, and green leafy vegetables. If you have severe bacterial overgrowth, introduce these foods slowly. Lightly cooking vegetables makes them easier to digest. Steam, sauté, or stir-fry instead of eating them raw.

Eat for Longevity

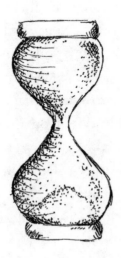

As soon as I turned 60, my focus on longevity intensified. I want to be as healthy as possible for as long as possible. I know many of you want the same. You want to live a long, active, engaged, healthy life and die young as late as possible.

LIFESPAN VS. HEALTHSPAN

Most people spend the last few decades of their lives (and sometimes more) with dysfunction, disability, and suffering from preventable and reversible ailments and on piles of pills. We are sicker than ever, and for the first time in history, our life expectancy is declining as our waistlines are expanding.

Advances in public health, surgery, and medicine are trying to extend our lifespan, but what about our health-span? Your lifespan is how long you live. Your healthspan is how many years you live a healthy, vibrant life. You want your healthspan to equal your lifespan.

The new science of longevity, based on the principles of functional medicine, is the science of health and restorative and regenerative medicine. It is not about just treating disease but about building resilience and vitality long-term. If you believe your genes are stacked against you, this is even more reason to double down on the science of creating health.

A large European study called EPIC found that incorporating four simple behaviors can dramatically reduce your risk of developing diseases of aging (Alzheimer's, diabetes, heart disease, and cancer). These include not smoking, exercising three and a half hours a week, eating a healthy diet, and maintaining a healthy weight. These four behaviors alone seemed to prevent 93 percent of diabetes cases, 81 percent of heart attacks, 50 percent of strokes, and 36 percent of all cancer cases.[30] No medication on earth can do that. You have to start with these foundational pillars.

Some say if you live longer, you will spend more time with chronic disease and disability, and in the hospital, increasing the burden on society and our health care system. Not true. Dr. James Fries' famous Stanford study found that if you kept your ideal weight, exercised, and didn't smoke, you were likely to live a long, healthy life and die painlessly, quickly, and cheaply.

UNIFIED THEORY OF AGING

The biggest cause of aging (and almost all age-related diseases) is something most doctors don't know how to diagnose or treat. It's also nearly 100 percent reversible. It's called *insulin resistance,* and it is at the root of heart disease, diabetes, cancer, and dementia. It also drives muscle loss as we age, leading to sarcopenia, which takes us down a rapid spiral into metabolic chaos and disability. Insulin resistance affects 88 percent of Americans to some degree. Ninety percent of people who have it are not diagnosed and have no clue they have it.

We focus on discovering the cure for this or that disease with this or that pill. It's like mopping the floor while the sink overflows. Turn off the faucet instead. This is a unified theory of aging. While many innovative therapies on the horizon can upgrade our biology and optimize aging, including stem cells, exosomes, peptides, hyperbaric oxygen, ozone, mitochondrial boosters, and supplements, unless you address insulin resistance first, you will be paddling upstream on a wild rushing river of disease and dysfunction.

How does insulin resistance happen? Simple: When you overeat starch (flour, pasta, bread, rice, and refined grains) and sugars in any form, your pancreas pumps out loads of insulin. Your cells become resistant to its effects, meaning that more and more insulin is required to keep your blood sugar normal. Until it can't, and then you get type 2 diabetes and a host of other problems, like increased belly fat, muscle loss, inflammation, hormonal imbalances, and brain damage. We eat an average of 152 pounds of sugar and

133 pounds of flour per person every year. Overall, processed food makes up 60 percent of our calories. No wonder half of Americans over age 60 have insulin resistance. It's happening to younger folks too. Kids as young as three years old now have type 2 diabetes. Fatty liver, formerly found only in older patients or alcoholics, now has soda-guzzling teenagers on the liver transplant list. These kids are 17 going on 70.

Hacking your blood sugar and insulin is the best way to live a long healthy life. A prominent Harvard cardiologist once said that if you found a group of 100-year-olds with perfectly clean arteries, they would have one thing in common: They would be insulin-sensitive, and their cells would require very little insulin to manage blood sugar. Most doctors never check fasting insulin levels or levels after a sugar load. Want a perfect test of how you are aging? This is it.

The Pegan Diet is the perfect insulin-sensitizing diet. For some of you already down the road of poor metabolic health, it may be critical to fix your metabolism by eliminating all starch and sugar for a few months or even a year. Over time, removing these foods will make you insulin-sensitive and able to ease back into eating starchy veggies, fruits, beans, and whole grains.

In addition to cutting starch and sugar, it's critical to eat more good fats and protective, disease-fighting foods. The polyphenol-rich foods I've mentioned throughout this book help with DNA repair, promote stem cell production, reduce inflammation, enhance our immunity, and supercharge our mitochondria (our energy factories, essential for aging well).

PROTEIN MAKES YOU YOUTHFUL

As we age, we also lose muscle and gain fat, even if we don't change our weight. Think marbled rib eye vs. filet mignon. Muscle loss is both a cause of and the result of insulin resistance. Diet plays an enormous role in muscle health. Unless you get enough of the high-quality building blocks of muscle, namely protein, you can't build muscle, especially as you age. Study after study links healthy aging and the preservation of muscle mass with higher-protein diets. Meat works the best.[31] Then chicken, then fish. Beans are last on the list. Plant proteins must be supplemented with additional amino acids or combined with animal protein to ensure they build muscle. Exercise and intake of omega-3 fats just before your protein intake can also increase muscle synthesis.[32] Goat whey protein powder is a great alternative for those wanting to avoid cow dairy and meat.

Lastly, there are a few hacks for reversing the biochemical and metabolic features of aging that can reverse insulin resistance, lower inflammation, boost antioxidants, rejuvenate your mitochondria, boost your stem cell production, increase your cognitive function, build muscle, and more. They have nothing to do with what you eat but everything to do with when you eat. As we reviewed in Principle 13, time-restricted eating and intermittent fasting and caloric restriction are proven ways to activate nearly every anti-aging mechanism in your body. Work with a practitioner to see if these tools are right for you. Start by incorporating at least a 12-hour window between dinner and breakfast.

No matter how old you are, you should be focused on longevity and maintaining strength, vitality, and energy.

PRINCIPLE 16 TAKEAWAYS

1. **Focus on fixing insulin resistance.** A fasting blood sugar level of 100 to 125 mg/dL or a hemoglobin A1c between 5.7 and 6.5 percent is considered prediabetes. Ideal blood sugar is 70 to 85 mg/dL. Ask your doctor to test your fasting insulin, which should be less than 5 μIU/dL, and 1- and 2-hour levels after a 75gm glucose load, which should be less than 30 μIU/dL. Your doctor may not be used to ordering this, but if you suspect you are not in tip-top metabolic health, insist on this test. If your markers are abnormal, take action now. Remove all sugars and refined starches from your diet, including bread, pasta, rice, and potatoes. Stress also causes insulin resistance, so learn to chill with meditation, yoga, and other relaxation techniques. Get moving and lifting. High-intensity interval training, short bursts of maximum-intensity exercise like sprinting, and muscle building with weights or your body weight are key to optimizing your metabolic health and preserving and building muscle.

2. **Focus on disease-fighting foods.** Follow the Pegan Diet and take extra care to incorporate loads of disease-fighting and protective foods. My favorites include green leafy vegetables and polyphenol-rich foods like cranberries, blackberries, wild or organic blueberries, pomegranate, and green tea; in fact, deeply colored plant foods should be the majority of your diet. The compounds in colorful plant foods are essential for longevity. Also include foods that help boost stem cells, repair DNA damage, and support immunity like turmeric, vitamin C–rich foods, cruciferous vegetables (like broccoli), and oysters.

3. **Build muscle.** I never liked the gym. I would rather be outside, but at 60, I bit the bullet, got a trainer, and started weight training. The gains in strength and muscle mass have surprised me. Even my back pain went away as my core got stronger. As we age, our risk of falling and injury increases. All of the

challenges that come with sarcopenia (muscle loss), including weaker muscles, poorer function, lower sex hormones, high insulin, worsening cholesterol, and high blood sugar, begin in your 30s and 40s. The only way to prevent this is to incorporate weight training. Find a trainer or ask someone at your gym for help. Start small and work your way up to heavier lifting. Bands and body-weight exercises also work well to build muscle.

4. **Incorporate time-restricted eating or intermittent fasting.** Do a 12-hour fast every day. Don't eat after dinner, and leave 12 hours until breakfast. And try a 16-hour fast twice a week or more if it works for you. I also recommend a 24-hour fast once a month, especially if you are overweight, overfat (thin on the outside but fat on the inside), or metabolically unhealthy.

If you start with these four habits, you are well on your way to better health. Remember, you can become young at any age!

Eat to Boost Mood

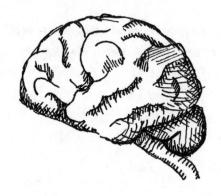

In 2020 we humans faced many obstacles—a pandemic; a flawed health care system; economic, social, and racial disparities. Many people lost jobs and businesses. Some dealt with tragic illnesses. Depression is now the fourth most common disease in the world and the number one cause of disability. We've been through a lot, and we need to support ourselves through this. Believe it or not, food can be a powerful tool to improve our mood and brain health; it can actually make us happier.

A growing body of science confirms the link between diet and brain health. Every single brain disorder—depression, anxiety, ADHD, autism, dementia, behavior problems, violence, and just plain old brain fog—is linked to diet, and often to the impact of our diet on our gut microbiome. Yet most people don't realize the profound connection between what we eat and our brain function. The body and the mind are a single, dynamic bidirectional system. What you do to one has an enormous impact on the other. You have to optimize all of the inputs and remove all of the bad influences.

It may be as simple as it was with my patient who had daily 3 p.m. panic attacks. He was a hard-driving New York financier, working all day and eating, drinking, and partying all night. He ate so much at night that he didn't eat again till late the next day. He had a big belly, insulin resistance, and wild swings in his blood sugar with hypoglycemia. Low blood sugar is a life-threatening emergency and turns on all the panic signals — increased heart rate, heavy breathing, sweating, and feeling like you are going to die, which you might unless you get some food. I had to get him to eat during the day and not at night. He also cut out sugar and starch and cut down on the alcohol — and instantly cured his panic attacks.

THE LINK BETWEEN NUTRITION, MOOD, AND BEHAVIOR

Whole new fields of research and academic departments such as nutritional psychiatry (at Harvard) and metabolic psychiatry (at Stanford) have emerged since I wrote *The UltraMind Solution* in 2008 about how the body affects the mind. Studies show that simply swapping out processed, sugary, starchy foods for whole foods (fruits, veggies, olive oil, nuts and seeds, legumes, and some meat — think Pegan) is effective in treating depression, in fact, 400 percent more effective than a typical Western diet.[33] Other studies show that kids with violent behavior transform when swapping out processed foods for whole foods. One study of violent juveniles found that simply giving children a vitamin and mineral supplement reduced violent acts by 91 percent compared to a control group.[34] Why were they violent? Their brains were starved of nutrients that regulate mood and behavior, including iron, magnesium, B_{12}, and folate.

Medical practice is slow to catch up to all the research, but you don't have to wait to feel better, calmer, and happier. What you eat today can boost your mood, improve your decision making, and make you more compassionate. Unfortunately, most of us don't take advantage of these truths. Instead, we go to our doctors, they tell us we have depression, but they don't tell us why. We're prescribed Prozac, but depression isn't a Prozac deficiency. Medication can be lifesaving for some (although for most with mild or moderate depression, antidepressants are not effective). But what about getting to the root cause?

Depression and anxiety are just the names given to a collection of symptoms, but many factors can cause each. Some people might have a B_{12} deficiency. Others might have an underactive or overactive thyroid. Still others could have low levels of vitamin D or gut dysfunction. New research clearly links depression and anxiety to brain inflammation. Rather than taking medication to suppress symptoms, the key to healing is to find the root cause. Why are you inflamed? The two biggest reasons are a processed, high-sugar, high-starch diet and imbalances in gut flora (also caused by diet, environmental toxins like glyphosate, and overuse of certain medications). Yes, use medication when necessary, but take other steps. Studies are clear. Diet and exercise often work better than medication, and all the side effects are good ones. Go to a functional medicine practitioner. And dig a little deeper.

EAT A BRAIN-BOOSTING DIET

The brain is resilient and can recover and heal under the right conditions. I have seen it over and over in thousands of my patients. We do many things that inflame our mood and our brains, including overeating sugar, refined carbs, and bad fats. We don't eat enough good fats, protective foods, and nutrients. We sleep too little, stay up too late, and stress too much. So how do we cool the fire within?

Start by cutting out refined sugars, processed carbohydrates, and artificial sweeteners. Make sure your blood sugar is balanced. This means eating during the day and not late into the night. Don't skip meals if you suspect you have blood sugar imbalances. Have you ever skipped a meal and felt wired and tired, with heart palpitations, dizziness, and loss of focus? Your body thinks you're dying. Make time to prepare balanced meals for breakfast, lunch, and dinner. Get a healthy dose of protein, whole food carbohydrates, and fats at every meal. Eating good fats helps cut cravings and prevents blood sugar crashes. Consider avoiding alcohol and heavily caffeinated beverages. If you do time-restricted eating, you need to be sure you have enough slow-burning fuels like fat and protein in your diet.

When it comes to brain disorders (anxiety, depression, memory loss, ADHD), nutritional deficiencies are the first place I look. A deficiency in any essential nutrient can create challenging symptoms, so it's important to work with a practitioner to get comprehensive blood work. The most common deficiencies I see related to brain disorders include omega-3 fats, magnesium, vitamin D, zinc, selenium, and B vitamins. Omega-3 fats, in particular, are critical for brain health. Sixty percent of your brain is made of DHA, an essential anti-inflammatory omega-3 fatty acid. If your brain is on fire, you're likely fat-deficient. Omega-3 fats form the basic structure of your cell membranes. If you don't have healthy cell membranes, your body's messenger molecules won't be able to communicate, and your health will suffer.

If you have symptoms of depression, anxiety, a mood disorder, irritability, or ADHD, you must check for nutritional deficiencies. I find that nine out of ten times, patients with these symptoms are deficient in at least one critical nutrient.

In the meantime, follow the Pegan Diet. Eat loads of veggies, some fruit (especially the low-sugar, nutrient-dense ones), whole grains (not flours), nuts and seeds, low-starch beans and legumes, and some high-quality meat, poultry, and fish. Focus on brain foods that have been shown to impact mood and reduce symptoms of depression and anxiety—foods rich in omega-3s, zinc, magnesium, vitamin D, antioxidants, and B vitamins.

Here are my favorite mood-boosting foods.

Food	Brain Benefits
Fatty fish and seafood like salmon and oysters	Fish is brain food. Consumption of the omega-3 fats in fish (EPA and DHA) has been linked to lower rates of depression and other brain disorders.
	Oysters contain a healthy dose of B_{12}, zinc, and omega-3 fats, making them one of my favorite brain foods.
Berries	Anthocyanins give berries their deep purple and blue color and have been shown to reduce depressive symptoms and boost cognitive function. I try to have either blueberries or blackberries every day.
Fiber-rich foods and fermented foods	They call the gut the second brain. To honor and optimize the connection between the gut and the brain, focus on gut-healing foods, including green leafy vegetables and fermented foods like sauerkraut.
Green tea	The phenolic content of green tea can reduce depressive symptoms. If you're looking for a polyphenol punch, enjoy a cup of green tea daily.
Nuts and seeds	Nuts and seeds contain tryptophan, the precursor to serotonin, which is our happy neurotransmitter. Tryptophan is also the precursor of melatonin, our sleepy hormone, which helps us get deep, restful sleep at night — critical for brain health!

If you suspect a deeper issue might be causing your mood disorder, for instance, nutrient deficiencies or an autoimmune condition, work with a licensed therapist or psychiatrist and a functional medicine practitioner to get to the root of your symptoms. It's humbling and inspiring to see patients bounce back from years of depression and anxiety after some detective work and tweaks.

PRINCIPLE 17 TAKEAWAYS

1. **Balance your blood sugar.** Don't skip meals, and eat a palm-size portion of protein, healthy fats, and plant foods with every meal. Imbalanced blood sugar alone is enough to make someone feel depressed, anxious, forgetful, and scattered.
2. **Eat brain-boosting foods.** Focus on fats from fish, berries, fiber-rich foods, nuts and seeds, and green tea if you can tolerate caffeine.
3. **Dig deeper.** Work with a practitioner to figure out if you have nutritional deficiencies, which are common with brain disorders.
4. **Consider supplementing with a good multivitamin** that includes B_6, folate, and B_{12}, and also consider taking vitamin D, magnesium, and omega-3 fats.

Make Healthy Eating Affordable

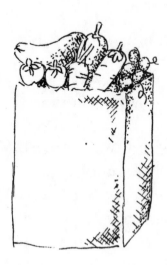

The prevailing myth is that eating well is expensive, inconvenient, and elitist, takes too much time, and is hard to do. The food industry encourages and even propagates this myth. Food manufacturers lure us into eating cheap and convenient food. Remember that McDonald's ad? "You deserve a break today!" Don't believe it. This myth keeps us buying fast food and packaged junk foods for convenience. The result—chronic disease, disability, and dependency on piles of pills. Hardly convenient or cheap.

Yes, processed food provides cheap calories. However, if you calculate the value of food based on nutrient density, not calories, then a bag of Cheetos would cost a fortune, and beans or collard greens or even a grass-fed steak would be cheap. There are no nutrients in Cheetos, but an abundance of vitamins, minerals, fiber, protein, and phytonutrients in whole plant and animal foods.

One day it will be significantly cheaper to eat well, but it is still possible to eat a real food diet on a budget.

IS A HEALTHY DIET REALLY THAT EXPENSIVE?

Studies show that a healthy diet costs around $1 to $2 more per day than the Standard American Diet.[35] Some studies show it can cost as little as 50 extra cents a day to improve the quality of your diet. When you include the real cost of cheap processed foods, eating real, whole foods is a far less expensive choice for our bodies and wallets. I'm still surprised when I hear people say that two avocados for $5 is too expensive, but then they load up on fast food meals for the whole family and coffee from Starbucks every day. While it might seem "cheaper" in the moment, eating out adds up. A roast chicken, baked sweet potato, and salad for four is cheaper than dinner out. When you buy real, whole food and cook at home, eating well is manageable, affordable, and fun.

During the filming of the movie *Fed Up,* about the role of sugar and the food industry in our obesity crisis, I visited a family in South Carolina, in one of the worst food deserts in the country. Their family of five lived on food stamps and disability. They were sick and obese. At 42 years old, the father was already on dialysis for kidney failure from type 2 diabetes. The mother and one teenage son were severely obese. They were living on all of the "diet" processed foods. They didn't know how to cook, but together we cooked a meal from fresh, whole ingredients. I gave them one of my cookbooks and a guide called *Good Food on a Tight Budget* from EWG (Environmental Working Group) on how to eat well for you, your wallet, and the planet, and they lost 200 pounds as a family. The 16-year-old son eventually lost 138 pounds and is now in medical school.

MAKE YOUR DOLLAR COUNT

When I was in residency, I supported my family of four on a salary of $27,000 a year. I shopped at discount stores, bought in bulk, and used real, fresh ingredients. We cooked delicious, homemade, healthy meals most nights of the week. Even if time and money are not on your side, you can still eat healthy whole foods. I'll never forget the importance of learning to eat well on a budget and continue to implement these strategies today. Here are my tips on eating well for less.

First, skip processed food. Processed, packaged foods are more expensive than fresh, whole foods. For $8 you can buy a frozen prepared meal for one person. For just a little more money (or sometimes less), you can make the same meal with better ingredients for the whole family. Fruits and veggies pack a lot of nutrients for little cost. Remember, fill 75 percent of your plate with non-starchy vegetables. You can also choose cheaper vegetables if you need to. Cabbage, carrots, beets, greens, onions, and sweet potatoes are very cheap, for example.

Buy ugly vegetables that would otherwise end up in landfills direct from farmers or Misfits or Imperfect Foods. Join your local CSA (community-supported agriculture) program and get a low-cost box of organic veggies and fruit weekly right from your local farms. Also eat whole grains and beans. They are among the most nutrient-dense and cheapest foods available. Meals for the family of beans or lentils and brown or wild rice won't break the bank. Add some broccoli or other greens, and you've got a nutritious and inexpensive meal. If you eat meat, source organic, pasture-raised, grass-fed, or regenerative animal products online and choose cheaper cuts. Check out Thrive Market, Butcher Box, and Mariposa Ranch. Get a freezer. Buy a cow share or half a cow. If you do that, the average cost per pound of regenerative meat is $8, or $2 for a 4-ounce serving—less cost per serving than a Big Mac, which is $3.99 for 3.2 ounces of meat (or, rather, a meatlike substance)!

Next, track where your money goes. You might be surprised to learn that your daily coffee at Starbucks or weekly happy hours add up. I'm sure many of you have learned that you can save money and have fun eating and hosting at home in the age of COVID-19. I also recommend keeping affordable staples on hand, such as extra virgin olive oil, avocado oil, vinegars, sea salt, pepper, spices, condiments, nut butters, nut milk, and frozen fruit. You can order staples online. New online stores like Thrive Market carry high-quality organic staples at 25 to 50 percent off retail prices. Once you become a member, you'll have direct access to wholesale prices on more than 3,000 healthy organic foods and products with fast shipping directly to your door. I get all of my staples like almond butter, turmeric, sea salt, and avocado oil online. Discount stores like Trader Joe's, Costco, Walmart, and Sam's Club also carry vegetables, clean meat, fruits, nuts, beans, fish, and staples like olive oil for significantly lower prices.

Another tip for keeping healthy eating affordable is to learn the Dirty Dozen and Clean Fifteen. Not everyone has the budget to buy 100 percent organic, but the more you can, the more you will avoid GMOs, pesticides, and glyphosate, and improve your health. See Principle 2 for more information on the Dirty Dozen (the most contaminated fruits and veggies) and the Clean Fifteen (the least contaminated), and buy accordingly.

When I was in residency and short on time and money, I would make the same meals every week. I call this the Master Five principle. You master five simple dinner meals that you can revisit when you get busy or money gets tight. Have the ingredients available at home so you don't get stuck eating food that doesn't make you feel good. This takes planning but is well worth it. In the recipes section, I've included five of my favorite meals to make on a budget. Just look for "Master Five" in the recipe description. You can also batch-cook and freeze meals. I batch-cook things like quinoa or brown rice. Sometimes I roast a whole chicken, and I can use it for at least two or three meals. I also recommend making large batches of soups or smoothies and freezing them. If you buy a bunch of meat, freeze everything you won't use right away to avoid food waste.

Before you go to the grocery, I highly recommend planning your meals. Money and time are wasted in wandering around aimlessly at the grocery store. Take 30 minutes before you shop to think about what you need for the week. Plan out breakfast, lunch, and dinner, at least for a few days at a time. Once you know what you need, you'll spend less money, and you won't pick up foods that might go to waste.

Remember, it is possible and not hard to eat healthy whole foods without breaking the bank. I did it, and with a few tips and some careful planning, you can do it too.

PRINCIPLE 18 TAKEAWAYS

1. **Stick to real, whole foods.** Processed and packaged foods will cost you more in the long run in terms of poor health and medical bills. If you stick to vegetables, fruits, beans, whole grains, and some high-quality animal foods, you'll save money.
2. **Take time to plan your meals and track your spending habits.** These two habits are underrated when it comes to saving money on food. Master five recipes that are affordable and that you can revisit every week.
3. **Shop online and at discount stores.** Check out Walmart, Costco, Trader Joe's, and Thrive Market. Join a CSA (community-supported agriculture) program to get farm fresh local food. If you're looking for more guidance on saving while eating well, use guides such as *Good Food on a Tight Budget* (ewg.org) to source the best foods at the best prices.

Feed Your Kids What You Eat

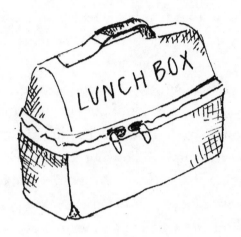

Raising healthy eaters starts early—very early. Epigenetics, how our genes get tagged or programmed by our environment for health or disease, begins in the womb. If a mother eats sugar and crap, the baby's genes get programmed for obesity, heart disease, diabetes, and even cancer. Starting early is vital in shaping biology and dietary preferences. Kids' food and kids' meals are a food industry invention. Happy Meals are anything but happy!

BUILDING HEALTHY HABITS TOGETHER

Over 30 years ago, when I became a father, I was determined to raise healthy eaters. We grew a garden. My daughter picked the eggplant early, wondering why it wouldn't crack! When she was three years old, she binged on Brussels sprouts. My kids got in the kitchen making food (and a mess) before they could even talk. I was a busy resident doctor working up to 80 hours a week, but family meals of real, whole food were always a priority.

Studies show that families who cook and eat together build healthy habits together. They're more likely to eat vegetables, and cooking together can positively benefit social intelligence, self-esteem, and academic performance. Cooking together reduces the risk of obesity and eating disorders and makes kids happier. Instilling healthy lifelong behaviors is best done by example. Take your kids food shopping and make cooking a fun activity. We used a cookbook called *Pretend Soup* with sixty-five kid-friendly recipes made from whole foods. Eating wholesome meals is about more than modeling sound nutrition; it's about family unity, connectedness, ritual, identity, and meaning. Children, even more than adults, enjoy and require routine. Shopping, cooking, and family meals can be an essential part of that routine.

It is not unusual to find families who prepare different meals for each family member, mostly from a box or package, each made in a different factory, eaten in under 20 minutes while watching television or distracted by smartphones. If there are food allergies, that's understandable, but my own house was not a restaurant. There were two things on the menu when the kids were growing up: take it or leave it.

Kids should eat what you eat, for the most part. Spicy foods and complex flavors and textures can be introduced slowly, but everyone can and should eat real, whole foods at any age. It's essential to set realistic boundaries about food choices and mealtimes. You provide the what, where, and when, and your child decides the if and how much. You don't have to force them to eat. It's okay if, in the beginning, your children are a little reluctant. Give them some time, and they'll slowly start to get curious about what you're eating. Or you can try my mother's approach, one she used on my sister when she didn't want eggs for breakfast. She didn't force her to eat them, but she gave her the same eggs for lunch, then for dinner, until she ate them. From then on, my sister ate what was in front of her.

Involve your kids in meal planning, grocery shopping, preparing, cooking (when they're old enough), serving, and cleaning up. Put on good music and make meal prep and mealtimes pleasant, relaxed, and fun—a time to come together as a family. Engage your children in conversation, and stay positive. Eating while stressed is not good for digestion, absorption, or metabolism. Similarly, don't use food to reward or punish children. Food is nourishment, and using it for anything else can create disordered eating as the child gets older.

It's also important to know when to be flexible. During holidays and birthdays, be easy on yourself and on your kids when they want the occasional indulgence. When they're sick, don't give in to the allure of comforting them with sugary treats. When they are healthy, they will thank you. Trust your young children to be naturally attuned to their hunger and satiety levels. Starting with and sticking with unprocessed whole foods sets them up for success long-term. Even if they rebel as teenagers, they will come back to what they learned as kids about healthy eating.

Now that we've covered setting up healthy habits, let's talk about how to feed your kids' bodies and brains!

HOW TO FEED YOUR KIDS

When your baby is ready to eat solid foods at about six months (this varies, depending on the child), make sure you take it slow and simple. Use one new food at a time. I recommend waiting three to five days before introducing another new food to observe any reactions or sensitivities. Stop a food immediately if your child responds poorly or shows symptoms of a food allergy.

Next, introduce vegetables and fruits before trying grains. Veggies and fruits are a bit easier on the digestive system. Mashed avocado is a great choice. If you want to try grains, try hypoallergenic ones like quinoa or brown rice. You can also puree or mash cooked food with a little bit of breast milk. This is a way of making your own baby food. Do you think our hunter-gatherer ancestors had Gerber's? Make homemade baby food safely by sterilizing equipment, labeling food with dates, discarding leftovers after three days, and properly storing labeled food in sterile containers in the refrigerator or freezer.

As your baby becomes a toddler, you can expand her diet. Try chopped cooked vegetables. Some great options are carrots, squash, and sweet potatoes. Mix in slightly bitter ones with the sweeter ones. Tiny chunks of fruit are also a great option, as are beans, peas, and lentils. Include whole, gluten-free grains like millet, quinoa, brown rice, or amaranth. For protein, try small chunks of fish, poultry, meat, tofu, or ground meat.

Most kids' food on the market today is riddled with artificial ingredients and sugars. My recommendation is to limit all refined sweeteners, candy, and even juices. Give your kids fruit for dessert instead. You can also hide veggies in homemade muffins, smoothies, and treats. Squash, carrots, sweet potatoes, and even spinach work well in baked goods. Soups, sauces, dips, spreads, and smoothies are also ways to get those vegetables in.

When it comes to dairy, I recommend avoiding all milk, cheese, and other dairy products until at least two years of age. Studies show that premature dairy intake can lead to allergies, respiratory infections, and weakened immunity. Goat or sheep products may be better tolerated. Start with sheep yogurt. Use only grass-fed dairy products. If you want to try cow dairy, find products from A2 cows.

As your kids get older, let them choose foods and plan meals with you. The more involved they are, the more likely they will be to experiment with various foods and flavors. Growing bodies need a healthy balance of nutrient-dense foods. Your kids can follow the Pegan Diet as long as they are not limiting calories. If your kids love pasta, try lentil or chickpea pasta. If they love pizza, make your own at home, using real ingredients. Try cauliflower crust. If they love fries, try sweet potato fries in your oven. If they love milkshakes, blend frozen fruit with non-dairy milk. There are plenty of healthy recipes for the whole family in this book.

PRINCIPLE 19 TAKEAWAYS

1. **Feed kids what you eat.** Your kids should eat what you eat. They do not need to eat off the kids' menu. Look at what kids in other countries (like Japan and France) eat for school lunches compared to school lunches in America. You'll be shocked.

2. **Start babies at six months with mashed fruits and veggies.** Avocado is one of the best first foods for babies. You can make your own baby food at home without all of the funky ingredients.

3. **Involve your toddlers and older kids in meal prep and planning.** Make grocery shopping, cooking, and mealtimes fun and positive. The more kids engage in food prep and food choices, the healthier they will be.

4. **Bad food creates bad behavior and impairs intellectual development.** Studies show what we eat influences our mood, behavior, and academic performance. Whole foods, rich in vitamins, minerals, fiber, good fats, and phytonutrients, can make kids less violent and improve behavior and grades. Sometimes kids need a little extra nutritional support. Talk to your pediatrician about incorporating an age-appropriate multivitamin, fish oil, and vitamin D.

5. **Feed kids brain food.** Some of my favorite foods for building healthy brain function include eggs, small fatty fish, greens, nuts and seeds, and berries. Healthy fats, especially omega-3 fats, are necessary for building a resilient brain.

6. **Eat Pegan with your kids.** As kids get older, encourage them to follow the Pegan Principles.

Make Healthy Habits Stick

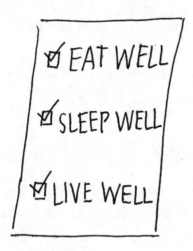

If you picked up this book, you likely care about eating well and living a healthy lifestyle, but caring and doing are different things. Information is often not enough. How do we shift our habits and create new ones?

Thankfully there is so much emerging science about behavior change. Understanding how to make, and sustain, change means identifying all of the steps between the intention and the behavior change and applying them. Our lifestyle choices, driven by our behavior, account for over half of the risk of early death. What we do every single day matters. Just like a marriage or a new skill, good health requires work. That work is personal, and it looks a bit different for everyone, but effort is needed. If you want to be healthy, you have to make that choice every single day and take action. Most of my life I focused on designing a healthy lifestyle; but still, to this day, I have to prioritize exercise, meditation, sleep, and cooking. Some days it feels effortless, and other days I would rather binge-watch Netflix with my wife. However, it does get easier, especially when you start to reap the benefits. Small steps and daily choices make a huge difference. One patient did not want to cut out her Doritos but decided to eat one less chip a day until she ate no more chips.

THREE STEPS TO MAKING LASTING CHANGE

The first step in creating optimal health is to know your "why." Why do you want to be healthy? My why is simple. I want to be full of energy, focus, and strength to live fully every day and do whatever I want without restriction. I want to dance all night, climb a mountain, learn a new language, and play sports. I want to keep my brain sharp. I have so many books I still want to read (and write). Most importantly, I want to be fully present for those I love and for my life's work and purpose. Identify your motivation. Do you want to have a baby and set that baby up for a healthy life? Do you want to boost your brain health because of work or school? Do you want to play sports, go for long hikes, and swim in oceans? Being healthy is not just about preventing disease; it's about living a life of vitality and energy. It's about getting to do what you love every single day.

After you identify your "why," enlist help. At the Cleveland Clinic Center for Functional Medicine, we implement group programs that often lead to more rapid and successful outcomes than individual appointments. One of my patients, Janice, was struggling with heart failure, type 2 diabetes, coronary artery disease, kidney failure, fatty liver, and low thyroid function, and she was on loads of medications to "manage" her illnesses. She saw so many different specialists who put her on different low-calorie, low-sodium diets, and nothing seemed to work. With the help of our Functioning for Life group program, she was able to get off of her insulin in three days. Her blood sugar, blood pressure, and cholesterol eventually normalized, and she lost more than 100 pounds. Her liver and kidney function returned to normal, and she even reversed her congestive heart failure. Her story sounds miraculous, but it isn't. It combines the science of food as medicine with the science of behavior change. Getting healthy, it turns out, is a team sport.

The Functioning for Life program is a 10-week group medical visit supported by doctors, nutritionists, health coaches, and behavioral therapists. Most participants report that this group effort is the critical missing piece to achieve lasting success. Human behavior is not isolated to our solitary habits; our social environment influences our behavior. As it turns out, noncommunicable diseases are very communicable. You are more likely to be overweight if your friends are overweight than if your family is overweight. If you have friends who are going to yoga and drinking green juice, you're more likely to do the same. If you have friends who are eating pizza and burgers and going to happy hour every night, you're more likely to live that way too. One of the critical elements in behavior change is your social circle. I don't want you to ditch your old friends (well, maybe some of them if they don't support your health journey). But if you don't have healthy friends, find some. If you don't know where to start, follow the advice of my friend Lewis Howes, who says, "Go where people grow."

Where do people better themselves? Yoga studios, fitness studios, healthy cafés and juice bars, bookstores. One of the best places to connect with like-minded folks is online. My 10-Day Reset has a supportive online Facebook group, where people have built friendships, shared recipes, and more. You can find more information in the Resources section on page 245.

Friend power is so much more powerful than willpower. If you have people cheering you on, holding you accountable, and walking the walk with you, you're much more likely to make positive changes. People who make New Year's resolutions are more likely to stick to them two or even six years later when they have social support. Don't go it alone. Enlist the help of at least one friend. Every body needs a buddy.

If you're having a tough time making lasting changes, start small. Sometimes we jump into a full-blown dietary overhaul, putting too much pressure on ourselves, and then we end up cheating, feeling guilty and ashamed—feelings that are not good for your mental or physical health (more on this in the next principle). In my practice, we meet people where they are. We start by incorporating small swaps. Instead of a carb-heavy breakfast like a muffin or a bagel, try a breakfast smoothie (you can find some in the recipes section). You can also try to swap the breadbasket for a side of vegetables, and swap soda for water. These simple swaps add up, and they are not overwhelming. We typically over-estimate what we can do in a day and underestimate what we can do in a year. Don't pack it all in right away. Start small, and soon enough, healthy eating and living will be like second nature.

PRINCIPLE 20 TAKEAWAYS

1. **Make your choice every single day and identify your "why."** Why is optimal health important to you? "Why" is more important than "how" and "what." Use this "why" as the guiding light that will keep you focused on your goals. Think of your "why" every single morning. I recommend printing it out and putting it in your kitchen, bedroom, or office. It's easy to let yesterday's motivation fall by the wayside. Think of your goals often: Keep a journal, and schedule time during the day to work toward them.

2. **Use friend power.** Don't underestimate the ability of a group of people or even one person to support you. Find people who want to get healthy or who have achieved what you want to achieve. If your family and friends are not on board, tell them that you need this time to take care of your health, and that you hope they will support your decisions. Find supportive friends and a tribe that will cheer you on. You can always look to the 10-Day Reset Facebook community.

3. **Start small.** You don't have to go dairy-free, sugar-free, gluten-free, or run 10 miles a day overnight. Start where you feel comfortable and build up slowly. Start substituting sugar-laden treats with fruit. Try adding more veggies to each meal. Try a smoothie for breakfast. Take a 10-minute walk. Do one push-up. When you feel less stress and more joy around

positive changes, you'll up-level your biology and reinforce these healthy habits. Honestly, I hated weight training. It hurt. It wasn't fun. The gym smelled. I started slowly and now I love it, and the payoff in terms of my strength and well-being makes it fun and easy!

4. **Study habit change.** Learn about science-based behavioral strategies from experts like B. J. Fogg from Stanford University in his book *Tiny Habits: The Small Changes That Change Everything,* or Charles Duhigg in his book *The Power of Habit: Why We Do What We Do in Life and Business.*

Start the Pegan Diet Today

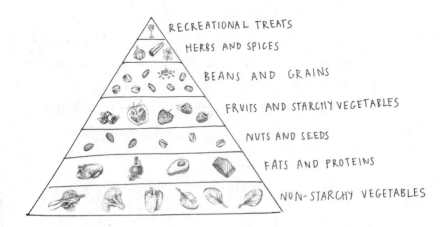

I've packed a lot of information into the last twenty principles—strategies for gut health, brain health, longevity, and more. We are inundated with an overwhelming amount of information about food and nutrition. Figuring out what to eat should be simple. We all just want to know "How do I get started?" My mission is to provide a road map for people to take control of their health. It is designed to be easy to implement, something you can start today. We all deserve an operating manual for our bodies and our health. The Pegan Diet is that manual. This principle synthesizes the key information you need to kick-start your health using the foundational rules of the Pegan Diet. Here's how to start the Pegan Diet.

ASK YOURSELF, *DID GOD (OR NATURE) MAKE THIS? OR DID MAN MAKE IT?*

The perfect diet has one hard rule: Eat real food, not food-like substances. When I say real food, I mean foods without labels or with ingredients you can recognize and pronounce—food that has barely changed from the field to your fork. Think heirloom organic corn on the cob instead of high-fructose corn syrup, whole grains instead of whole wheat bread, pasture-raised chicken instead of chicken nuggets. Did God make a doughnut? Nope. Did God make an apple? Yes. Even a five-year-old can understand that.

TRY TO AVOID FOODS WITH LABELS

There are some exceptions to this rule, of course. Things like olive oil and nut butter have a label, but for the most part, stick with foods that don't require a label. A bag of chips has a label. A bag of avocados does not. If the ingredients are things you would have in your kitchen, the food may be fine. Canned tomatoes have water, tomatoes, and salt. Also, avoid foods with a health claim on the label. "All-Natural" and "Heart-Healthy" are written only on processed food-like substances. They are not printed on a bushel of kale or broccoli. Health claims trick people. Gluten-free potato chips are not a health food. You don't need a health claim to tell you that whole fruits and veggies are good for you.

DON'T EAT THINGS WITH INGREDIENTS YOU CAN'T PRONOUNCE OR WOULDN'T HAVE IN YOUR CUPBOARD OR FRIDGE

Additives, preservatives, dyes, MSG, artificial sweeteners, and other "Frankenchemicals" are ingredients that you wouldn't cook with at home, so why purchase foods containing these chemicals? Avoid all funky ingredients that sound more like science experiments than actual food. Also avoid GMO foods. We still don't understand how GMOs affect human health. And they usually come with higher levels of glyphosate (weed killer) and pesticides. Why take the risk?

SHOP THE PERIPHERY OF THE GROCERY STORE

The easiest way to make sure you're buying real foods is to shop the outer aisles of the grocery store. This is where you'll find fresh food like vegetables, fruits, meat, poultry, eggs, and fish. The middle aisles tend to contain mostly processed food-like substances, so spend more time in the outer aisles. The exception is foods like nuts, seeds, and oils, often found in the middle aisles.

EAT MOSTLY PLANTS

When you eat plants, you benefit from the array of beneficial, disease-fighting compounds that they carry. Fill 75 percent of your plate (by volume) with colorful plant foods. Adding two cups of green leafy vegetables is an easy way to up your plant intake. Eat broccoli, bok choy, arugula, tomatoes, peppers, kale, and all of the other plants discussed in Principles 2 and 3. Limit starchy vegetables to half a cup per day, or even less (half a cup per day up to three times a week) if you have prediabetes or are diabetic. Eat low-glycemic fruits like berries and kiwi—limit them to half a cup per day or one piece of fruit per day.

USE MEAT AS A CONDIMENT, OR "CONDI-MEAT"

Remember, the Pegan Diet is not a meat-heavy diet. You need a palm-size amount of protein for each meal (vegetarian or meat protein). Have grass-fed meat, organic and ideally pasture-raised poultry or eggs, fatty fish, or non-GMO and organic tofu or tempeh or low-starch beans and lentils. Vegetables should take center stage, and meat should be the side dish. I usually have about 4 to 6 ounces of animal protein twice a day max.

EAT FAT WITH EVERY MEAL

As you've learned, fat is essential for the functioning of a healthy body—it is one of the body's most basic building blocks. The average person is made up of between 15 and 30 percent fat! Contrary to misguided advice offered over the last 30-plus years, the right fats are needed for healthy skin, cells, brain functioning, fertility, and more. The wrong fats (refined vegetable oils like canola, safflower, and soybean oil) are deadly. Focus on 3 to 5 servings of healthy fats a day like avocado, nuts and seeds, and olive oil. One serving of fat is a tablespoon of olive oil or half an avocado.

INCLUDE SPECIAL SUPERFOODS

A food qualifies as a superfood if it is nutritionally dense. Prioritize all the superfoods that I've discussed throughout this book, including colorful plant foods, grass-fed meat, and wild fatty fish. My favorite superfoods include berries, green tea, wild salmon, anchovies, grass-fed meat, goat yogurt, broccoli, black rice, and leafy greens like broccoli. All of the powerful phytochemicals in these foods can help prevent and fight disease and feed your body with healing information.

AVOID DAIRY (MOSTLY)

There's a reason Paleo and vegan folks avoid dairy. Few can tolerate it, and for most, it can contribute to acne, congestion, obesity, diabetes, heart disease, and osteoporosis. If you like dairy, stick with nutritionally dense dairy, like butter, ghee, and goat and sheep yogurt and cheese.

STICK TO GLUTEN-FREE, WHOLE FORMS OF GRAINS

We don't need grains, but that doesn't mean they're all terrible for us. Grains can increase your blood sugar, especially if they are in the form of flours. I do not recommend flour-based products or gluten on a regular basis. Our modern forms of wheat and gluten fuel inflammation, autoimmune disease, digestive disorders, and obesity. Heirloom gluten grains like einkorn wheat or heirloom rye or barley may be well tolerated by those who are not gluten-sensitive. But it is a good idea for most people to do a three-week 100 percent gluten-free trial followed by reintroduction to see how gluten affects them. Most have no idea how much better they can feel on a gluten-free diet.

A little bit of nut flour or grain-free alternatives are fine here and there, but stay away from grain-based flours. Stick with small portions (half a cup) of low-glycemic grains like black rice or quinoa. If you are prediabetic or diabetic, or have insulin resistance, belly fat, or an autoimmune disease, you might want to remove grains completely for three weeks and see how you feel.

EAT NUTS, SEEDS, AND LOW-STARCH BEANS

Nuts and seeds are a staple in the vegan diet. Beans are also great and a good source of fiber, protein, and minerals. But they do cause digestive problems for some, and if you have diabetes, a mostly bean diet can trigger spikes in blood sugar. Half a cup to one cup per day is fine for some. If you have insulin resistance, prediabetes, diabetes, or an autoimmune condition, you might benefit from removing beans temporarily. My overall advice is to stick to low-starch beans like black beans, lupini beans, and lentils. Nuts and seeds are some of my favorite superfoods. I have about a handful or two a day, including almonds, chia seeds, macadamia nuts, hemp seeds, and more. See a full list on page 168.

ENJOY PLEASURE FOODS, BUT DON'T MAKE THEM A DAILY HABIT

The Pegan Diet is not about perfection. We are all going to indulge in something at one point or another. The key is to prevent indulgences from becoming habits. Enjoy sugar (in all of its forms) on occasion or sparingly. When treats like pastries, wine, cocktails, beer, and so on become a daily habit they contribute to disease. Instead, enjoy recreational treats once in a while, and stick to the Pegan Diet 90 percent of the time. I keep my treats to a piece of dark chocolate a day, and a healthy homemade dessert once a week. A few times a month I'll have a glass of wine or a cocktail with friends. That's what works for me. Others can have a glass of wine or a cocktail up to three times a week and feel fine. When it comes to treats, make sure you're eating real, whole food treats, not an industrial science project designed to be addictive. And if you want something like cookies or pie, make it yourself from real ingredients. If you want French fries occasionally, make them yourself, or better yet, make baked fries with truffle oil and salt. Easy and delicious.

This way of eating helps regenerate your health and the health of the planet. The field of nutrition is complicated, and the truth is that no one way works for everyone's beliefs, preferences, and genetic makeup. The Pegan Diet is all about simple rules customized on the basis of your needs.

PRINCIPLE 21 TAKEAWAY

Eat a variety of colorful plant foods throughout the day. Eat a palm-size amount of animal- or plant-based protein per meal. Add a serving or two of healthy fats to each meal. Avoid foods with labels and ingredients that you can't pronounce. Avoid conventional dairy, gluten, and sugar. Don't be too hard on yourself. Here's a Pegan Diet cheat sheet.

Vegetables	Eat unlimited non-starchy vegetables: artichokes, asparagus, avocado, bean sprouts, broccoli, Brussels sprouts, cabbage, carrots, cauliflower, celery, cucumber, eggplant, garlic, ginger root, hearts of palm, kohlrabi, leafy greens, mushrooms, onions, peppers, radicchio, radish, rutabaga, seaweed, shallots, summer squash, tomatoes, turnips, zucchini.
	Limit starchy vegetables to ½ cup per day: yam, sweet potatoes, winter squash, pumpkin.
Fruit	Eat ½ cup of fruit or 1 piece of fruit per day. Focus on low-glycemic fruits such as blackberries, blueberries, cranberries, kiwi, lemons, limes, raspberries.
Animal protein	Eat 4 to 6 ounces of animal protein twice a day max: pasture-raised, hormone- and antibiotic-free chicken, eggs, turkey, duck, pheasant, Cornish game hen; grass-fed, pasture-raised lamb, beef, bison, venison, ostrich, deer, elk; anchovies, clams, cod, crab, flounder/sole, herring, small halibut, mussels, wild salmon, sardines, sable, shrimp, scallops, trout.
Nuts, seeds, beans, grains	Eat 1 to 2 handfuls of nuts and/or seeds daily.
	Nuts: almonds, Brazil nuts, cashews, hazelnuts, macadamia, pecans, pine nuts, pistachios, walnuts, raw cacao
	Seeds: chia, flax, hemp, pumpkin, sesame, sunflower
	Eat up to ½ cup of low-starch beans daily: green beans, green peas, lentils, lupini beans, miso, natto, non-GMO soy, tempeh, chickpeas, black beans, snap peas, snow peas.
	Eat up to ½ cup of whole grains daily: quinoa, black rice, brown rice, red rice, wild rice, teff, amaranth, buckwheat.
Dairy	Grass-fed butter, ghee, goat and sheep yogurt and cheese are fine in moderation.
Beverages	Drink purified water, herbal tea, seltzer, mineral water, green juices with just greens or a little bit of lemon.
	Coffee and caffeinated tea are okay if you don't get the jitters or have adverse reactions.
	Limit alcohol to 1 glass of wine or 1 cocktail up to 3 times a week.

Oil and condiments	For cooking, use grass-fed ghee; humanely raised tallow, lard, duck fat, chicken fat; organic avocado oil; or organic virgin coconut oil.
	For salads, use almond oil, flax oil, hemp oil, macadamia oil, extra virgin olive oil (also good for low or medium heat), sesame seed oil, tahini, walnut oil.
Sugar and sweeteners	Eat very small amounts of stevia, monk fruit, maple syrup, honey, date sugar, coconut sugar, or molasses. These should not be daily foods.

Cook the Pegan Way

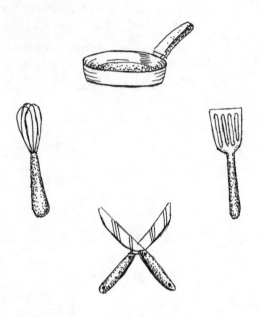

Cooking is a lost skill but the most important one for health and longevity (unless you have a personal chef!). We have now raised generations of Americans who don't know how to cook and spend more time watching cooking on television than actually cooking. Not only is cooking good for you; it's also a powerful way to drive change in our food system. You get to pick what you buy and where the food comes from, which influences the marketplace to produce better food. If everyone stopped buying soda, or factory-farmed meat, or food with high-fructose corn syrup, it would start a food revolution from farm to fork.

We have been trained to think that cooking is a burden,

drudgery, and time-consuming. Yet it is one of the most essential acts that make us human. Michael Pollan, in his book *Cooked,* says, "The decline of everyday home cooking doesn't only damage the health of our bodies and our land but also our families, our communities, and our sense of how our eating connects us to the world." Wendell Berry said that "eating is an agricultural act." It is also a political act, and so is cooking.

How do we end our current chronic disease epidemic and health care, environmental, and financial crises? We have to cook our way out. When we cook, we rebuild our communities, strengthen the bonds within our families, and nourish our bodies and souls. Cooking is also fun.

Remember, it's typically not the salt, sugar, or other ingredients that you add to your home-cooked meals that pose a problem. It's the salt, sugar, bad fats, and unpronounceable toxic ingredients that food companies add to their food that damage your health. Cooking is your way out of sickness, and your path to freedom from processed food and toward vibrant health and a happier life.

As I'm writing this, the entire world is sheltering in place because of COVID-19. Restaurants are closed, and most of us have little to no access to takeout. More people are cooking at home; in fact, nearly everyone must. My hope is that even though this is a tremendously difficult time, it brings everyone closer together and makes everyone more connected to their kitchens and to cooking.

Before we get to the recipes, let's cover some cooking basics to set you up for success.

HAVE FUN

If you view cooking as a burden, you probably won't get into the kitchen often. Instead, turn on the music, grab a loved one, stay calm, smile, and go with the flow. Pick fun recipes for dishes you love. Try new dishes. Once you learn how to cook from recipes, what order to add ingredients, which foods go best together, or how to use different spices, you'll be able to improvise and play a little. It's like learning to play a musical instrument. It doesn't have to be perfect. Make mistakes. Learn for next time.

PREPARE YOUR FRIDGE AND PANTRY

Keep basics on hand.

- Organic extra virgin olive oil for drizzling and low-temperature cooking.
- Avocado oil for high-temperature cooking.
- Salt and pepper. They are foundational for most recipes. I love Redmond Real Salt, a mineral salt from an ancient Utah seabed.
- Your favorite spices and herbs. My favorites are paprika, turmeric, cumin, coriander, cardamom, thyme, dill, rosemary, cinnamon, cayenne, chili powder, oregano, cloves, and mustard seeds. Spices help you go on a world food journey. Try Mexican one night, Thai another. How about Indian, Japanese, Moroccan, Greek, or Italian? It is the spices that make cuisines unique and provide a powerful medicinal healing punch along with the flavor.

- Add acids. I love lemon, lime, apple cider vinegar, and balsamic vinegar. You can make full salad dressings with just olive oil, an acid, and spices.
- Finally, get a basic set of kitchen tools. Mozart needed many instruments to make beautiful music. Get good knives, pots and pans, mixers, peelers, wooden spoons, and more. See my favorites in the Resources section on page 245.

LEARN TO COOK VEGGIES WELL

Learning to cook veggies properly can change your life. Most American vegetables end up as overcooked tasteless mush. People often claim they don't like Brussels sprouts or asparagus. My response is that they don't know how to prepare them properly. You first have to learn cooking basics and then experiment with flavors that you enjoy.

- **Sauté:** This is my favorite way to prepare vegetables. Heat a large sauté or frying pan over medium heat. Add 1 tablespoon of avocado oil, grass-fed butter, or ghee to the pan. When the oil shimmers, add the vegetables, allowing them to cook for about 2 to 5 minutes. If you want to take the flavors up a notch, first add some onion, garlic, and ginger and cook for 1 to 2 minutes. Vegetables like asparagus will cook in just 3 to 4 minutes. Sturdier vegetables like cauliflower will take a few minutes longer. Add a splash of water or a little mirin, a Japanese rice wine that makes everything taste good.
- **Steam:** Steamed vegetables are easy, fresh, crunchy, and nutrient-packed. I love to steam broccoli (or any

vegetable) and toss it with a mixture of extra virgin olive oil, lemon juice, a fresh-pressed garlic clove, and a little salt and pepper. Insert a steamer basket into a large pot. Fill the pot with several inches of water to just below the steamer rack. With the lid on, bring the water to a boil over medium–high heat. Add the vegetables to the steamer, cover, turn the heat down to medium, and steam until crisp-tender. Most vegetables take 2 to 5 minutes. Green ones should still be bright green. If they turn dark, they are overcooked.

- **Roast:** Preheat your oven to 425°F. Line a baking sheet with foil or parchment paper for easier cleanup. Toss your vegetables with olive oil, salt, pepper, and any other spices you like. Arrange the vegetables on the baking sheet and roast until the vegetables are crisp and tender. Asparagus usually takes about 5 to 10 minutes, but cauliflower and broccoli take about 20 to 30 minutes. Roasting carrots or other root vegetables might take about 40 minutes. You can add the veggies that need more time first, then throw in the quicker-cooking veggies later.

DON'T OVER- OR UNDERCOOK PROTEIN

Preparation is critical when it comes to cooking meat, poultry, and fish. You want to avoid under- and overcooking it. Raw poultry and meat are a hotbed of bacteria. High-temperature cooking leads to toxic compounds that can damage your health. I recommend getting a meat thermometer to measure temperature. Also, use medicinal spices in marinades to reduce inflammation.

- Meat will be done, depending on your preference, at an internal temperature from 130°F to 135°F for medium-rare, or 140°F to 145°F for medium-cooked steaks, roasts, and chops. Here's a great way to cook steak. If you're cooking steak on the stovetop, salt the steak about 30 minutes before you cook it. Heat up a pan (I like cast-iron pans for steaks). The steak will need only about 4 to 6 minutes on each side, depending on thickness. Cook until the desired temperature is reached. Season with your favorite spices and herbs.

- Ground meat and poultry should be cooked to 165°F. Heat a large pan with avocado oil over medium-high heat. Add the meat to the hot pan and break it into pieces using a spatula. Cook until browned.

- Bake your chicken until the internal temperature reaches 165°F. For baked chicken breasts, heat the oven to 350°F. Combine your favorite marinade in a bowl. I like garlic, olive oil, lemon juice, basil, and sea salt. Place the chicken breasts in the bowl, coat them with the marinade, and let them marinate for 15 minutes. Line your baking dish with parchment paper for easy cleanup. Place the chicken and extra marinade in the pan. Cook for about 30 minutes until the chicken reaches the desired temperature.

- Cook fish until it's about 145°F. Here's a way to cook the perfect salmon. Heat your pan over medium-high heat. While that's happening, season your salmon. Add avocado oil to the pan and place the fish skin side down. Let it cook for about 7 minutes. Don't touch it, as tempted as you might be. After 7 minutes, it'll be mostly cooked. Flip it over but be careful of the hot oil. Cook for an additional 2 minutes. At this point it should be perfect.

MASTER COOKING HACKS

You can master three things in one day. They include a smoothie, a salad, and a basic stir-fry. They are super easy and nutritious. You can swap in ingredients that you already have or try out new ones.

- **Simple smoothie:** Blend 8 ounces of unsweetened non-dairy milk (my favorite is Milkadamia), ½ cup of frozen berries, 1 handful of spinach or other leafy greens, 1 tablespoon of nut butter, and 1 tablespoon of flaxseeds or chia seeds. That's it—a perfect smoothie. You can add a scoop of my Pegan Shake for extra protein, fat, and fiber (getfarmacy.com/pegan).

- **Super easy salad:** To a salad bowl add 1 bunch of chopped greens (I like butter lettuce or arugula), as many non-starchy veggies as you like (peppers, cucumbers, radish, fennel, green onion, olives), a can of wild salmon or 2 to 6 ounces of chicken, 3 tablespoons of your favorite herbs and spices (parsley, cilantro, mint, basil), 2 tablespoons of extra virgin olive oil, and 1 to 2 tablespoons of lemon juice, balsamic vinegar, or apple cider vinegar. Toss everything together and serve!

- **Kitchen sink stir-fry:** Heat avocado oil in a large pan over medium heat. Add chopped onion and sauté for 2 to 3 minutes; then add chopped or pressed garlic, a little ginger, and 3 cups of chopped vegetables. Try fennel, leeks, carrots, zucchini, cauliflower, asparagus, onions, broccoli, or pretty much anything else. Add spices like paprika or cumin. Make it Asian with a little bit of toasted sesame oil, gluten-free tamari, and mirin. Cook for about 10 to 15 minutes or less. Top with lemon juice and fresh herbs like parsley or cilantro, and add salt to taste. Add your favorite protein like cooked ground meat or sliced chicken, beef, tempeh, or tofu.

I promise you that anyone can learn to love cooking, even if your only experience is heating TV dinners or toasting bread. Once you learn to appreciate flavors, let loose, and experiment in the kitchen, you'll be able to nourish your body and give joy and pleasure to those you love. Oh, and you'll also revolutionize your health.

The Pegan Diet is built on a foundation of eating and cooking real, whole food. I hope you incorporate the Pegan Principles in your life and discover the pleasure, joy, nourishment, and healing power of food. Remember, food is medicine. Your grocery store is your farmacy!

Next up are my favorite Pegan recipes, including breakfast, lunch, dinner, basics, drinks, sides, and more.

Let's get cooking!

Breakfast

Avocado Latke "Toast"

Serves: 4
Prep time: 35 minutes
Cook time: 40 minutes

Avocado toast has become so popular, but I'm never a fan of store-bought bread full of refined flour. For this healthier version, I layered yam latkes (potato pancakes) with a simple take on guacamole, a fresh fennel slaw, and a soft-boiled egg. Fennel is an underused vegetable rich in minerals and protective polyphenol antioxidants like rosmarinic acid, chlorogenic acid, and quercetin, with a unique slightly licorice flavor.

Yam Latkes

- 3 cups grated Japanese white yam (or any type of yam/sweet potato)
- ¾ cup grated white onion
- 1 small jalapeño, seeds and ribs removed, finely chopped (optional)
- ¼ cup plus 2 tablespoons ground flaxseed
- ½ teaspoon garlic powder
- ½ teaspoon black pepper
- ¼ cup avocado oil
- 3 pasture-raised egg whites, beaten

Fennel Slaw

1 large fennel bulb with fronds

10 fresh mint leaves, torn

2 tablespoons sundried tomatoes, chopped

1 small shallot, finely chopped

2 tablespoons fresh lemon juice

1 tablespoon extra virgin olive oil

⅛ teaspoon sea salt

¼ teaspoon black pepper

Smashed Avocado

1 large avocado, halved and pitted

½ cup fresh cilantro, tightly packed

Juice and zest of 1 lime

1 small jalapeño, seeds and ribs removed, finely chopped (optional)

1 tablespoon extra virgin olive oil

¼ teaspoon black pepper

Soft-Boiled Eggs

4 pasture-raised eggs

1. Preheat the oven to 375°F and line a baking sheet with parchment paper.
2. For the latkes: Add the grated yams and onion to a fine strainer and press to remove excess moisture. In a large bowl, mix the jalapeño (if using), ground flaxseed, garlic powder, pepper, avocado oil, and egg whites together. Add the yams and onions and mix well until combined.
3. Pack the mixture into a ¼-cup measuring cup and turn out each latke onto the sheet. Use your hands to flatten. You should have 8 latkes minimum. Bake for 15 minutes, flip, and bake for another 15 minutes until golden brown and crispy.

4. Prepare the salad by removing the stalks and fronds from the fennel bulb. Coarsely chop the fronds and thinly slice the stalks. Place in a large bowl. Using a mandoline, thinly slice the bulb, cutting it in half if necessary. Add the fennel to the bowl along with the torn mint and chopped sundried tomatoes.

5. In a separate small bowl, add the minced shallots, lemon juice, olive oil, salt, and pepper.

6. Prepare the smashed avocado by scooping the avocado into a small bowl and roughly mashing it. Add the cilantro, lime juice, lime zest, jalapeño (if using), olive oil, and pepper. Mix until combined but chunky.

7. To make the soft-boiled eggs, bring a large saucepan of water to a boil over medium-high heat. Using a slotted spoon, carefully lower the eggs into the water one at a time. Cook for exactly 6½ minutes, adjusting the heat to maintain a gentle boil. Transfer the eggs to a bowl of ice water and chill for 2 minutes. Once cooled, gently crack the eggs and peel.

8. Combine the fennel mixture with the dressing. Assemble the dish by layering one yam latke with smashed avocado, adding another latke, then a scoop of salad, and topping with an egg. Repeat to make 4 total and serve.

Nutritional Analysis Per Serving: Calories: 566, Fat: 36 g, Saturated Fat: 5 g, Cholesterol: 185 mg, Fiber: 13 g, Protein: 17 g, Carbohydrates: 47 g, Sodium: 309 mg

Morning Quinoa Berry Bake

Serves: 6
Prep time: 15 minutes plus 10 minutes to cool
Cook time: 1 hour

Some mornings just call for a warm, comforting bowl of baked goodness. This is that dish, complete with protein-rich quinoa, nuts, and seeds, and a variety of colorful sweet berries bursting with vitamin C and anti-aging phytochemicals. You can use any combination of berries you like for a total of 3 cups. Fresh is best, but frozen works too!

1 teaspoon avocado oil

1 cup sprouted white quinoa

1 medium zucchini

2 cups unsweetened nut milk

½ cup filtered water

Zest of 1 orange

2 teaspoons pure vanilla extract

1 teaspoon ground cinnamon

¼ teaspoon ground nutmeg

Pinch of sea salt

⅓ cup hulled hemp seeds

¼ cup ground flaxseed

2 tablespoons unsweetened shredded coconut

⅓ cup sweetener of choice (monk fruit, liquid maple sweetener, pure maple syrup, or raw honey, optional)

1 cup (about 8) strawberries, quartered

1 cup (about 15) blackberries, halved

½ cup raspberries

½ cup blueberries

¼ cup raw whole pecans

¼ cup raw sliced almonds

1. Preheat the oven to 350°F. Grease a 10½ x 7-inch oven-safe casserole dish with the avocado oil. Rinse the quinoa thoroughly and pour it into the dish, spreading evenly.

2. Using a box grater, shred the zucchini using the smallest side of the box. Using your hands, squeeze out the excess water. You should have 1 cup of shredded zucchini. Add to the casserole dish with the quinoa and stir together.

3. In a medium-size bowl, add the nut milk, water, zest, vanilla extract, cinnamon, nutmeg, salt, hemp seeds, flaxseed, shredded coconut, and sweetener of choice, if using. Mix well. Pour on top of the quinoa and zucchini and mix together.

4. Drop the berries into the casserole dish, spreading them evenly. Break up the pecans into small pieces and sprinkle with the sliced almonds. Using a spatula, press them gently into the liquid and flatten the surface.

5. Cover the dish and bake for 30 minutes. After 30 minutes, raise the oven temperature to 375°F and bake, uncovered, for 30 more minutes. The liquid should be absorbed and the quinoa golden and sticky.

6. When ready, remove from the oven and let cool for 10 minutes before serving. Store leftovers in the fridge for up to 4 days.

Nutritional Analysis Per Serving (without added sweetener): Calories: 307, Fat: 17 g, Saturated Fat: 2 g, Cholesterol: 0 mg, Fiber: 8 g, Protein: 11 g, Carbohydrates: 31 g, Sodium: 87 mg

Matcha Poppy Bread with Rose Water Glaze

Makes: 12 slices
Prep time: 20 minutes
Cook time: 30 to 35 minutes

This delicious grain-free loaf makes a unique breakfast or uplifting snack. Packed with antioxidants from matcha green tea powder and plenty of healthy monounsaturated fats from olive oil, it provides long-lasting energy. The glaze adds a sweet floral note with a hint of rose water. This bread is unlike any other and is sure to become a new family favorite.

Matcha Poppy Bread

½ cup extra virgin olive oil

2 large pasture-raised eggs

½ cup unsweetened almond milk

1½ teaspoons pure vanilla extract

2 tablespoons raw honey (optional)

2 tablespoons poppy seeds

1½ cups fine almond flour

¼ cup coconut flour

1½ tablespoons matcha powder

½ cup granulated monk fruit, for baking

½ teaspoon sea salt

1 teaspoon baking soda

Rose Water Glaze

¼ cup ghee or softened coconut oil

1 teaspoon rose water

1 teaspoon powdered monk fruit or raw honey

Optional Garnish

Powdered monk fruit
Raw sliced almonds
Edible dry rosebuds and rose petals

1. Preheat the oven to 350°F. Lightly grease an 8 x 4-inch loaf pan with olive oil and line the bottom with parchment paper.
2. In a medium-size bowl, whisk together the olive oil, eggs, almond milk, vanilla extract, honey (if using), and poppy seeds. Whisk well until fluffy. Set aside.
3. In a large bowl, sift together the almond flour, coconut flour, matcha powder, monk fruit, salt, and baking soda and stir to combine.
4. Add the wet ingredients to the dry ingredients, stirring well. Pour the batter into the prepared pan and use a spatula to smooth the top.
5. Bake for 30 to 35 minutes or until a toothpick inserted into the center comes out clean. Let cool in the pan for 10 minutes before turning the bread out of the pan.
6. Meanwhile, prepare the glaze by combining all the ingredients together in a small bowl.
7. If you choose to garnish, use a fine-mesh sieve to dust the bread with powdered monk fruit, then top with sliced almonds and edible rosebuds and petals. Serve slices warm or at room temperature with glaze on the side for dipping or drizzling.
8. Store leftovers wrapped well in the refrigerator for up to 3 days.

Nutritional Analysis Per Slice (using ghee, without honey): Calories: 217, Fat: 19 g, Saturated Fat: 5 g, Cholesterol: 42 mg, Fiber: 4 g, Protein: 5 g, Carbohydrates: 14 g, Sodium: 221 mg

CHAI PANCAKES WITH COCONUT WHIPPED CREAM

Makes: 14 (4-inch) pancakes
Prep time: 20 minutes
Cook time: 30 minutes

For those who like the occasional indulgent breakfast, this one is for you. But instead of refined flour and sugar, I use wholesome fiber- and nutrient-packed buckwheat and almond flours and monk fruit sweetener, which has zero glycemic load. So you can enjoy these guilt-free. Get creative and use whatever toppings you like; fresh figs are one of my personal favorites.

Coconut Whipped Cream

1 (14-ounce) can coconut cream, chilled in refrigerator overnight
⅓ cup powdered monk fruit

Chai Pancakes

2 large pasture-raised eggs
1½ cups unsweetened almond milk
2 teaspoons pure vanilla extract
¼ cup coconut oil, melted
3 tablespoons granulated monk fruit sweetener, for baking (optional)
¼ cup raw pecans, crushed
1 cup buckwheat flour
½ cup almond flour
1 teaspoon baking powder
½ teaspoon baking soda
¼ teaspoon sea salt
2 teaspoons ground cinnamon

¼ teaspoon ground cardamom
¼ teaspoon ground ginger
½ teaspoon ground cloves
½ teaspoon ground nutmeg

Garnish

Pure maple syrup (optional)
Fresh figs, sliced (optional)

1. Place a large mixing bowl in the refrigerator to make the coconut whipped cream in later. In another large bowl, beat together the eggs, almond milk, vanilla extract, 2 tablespoons of the coconut oil, and the monk fruit, if using. Beat until the eggs are fully incorporated and the mixture is fluffy. Fold in the crushed pecans.

2. In another large bowl, sift the buckwheat and almond flours, baking powder, baking soda, salt, 1½ teaspoons of the cinnamon, cardamom, ginger, cloves, and nutmeg. Slowly add the dry ingredients to the wet ingredients, stirring well until fully combined and no lumps remain.

3. Heat a large skillet over medium heat. When the pan is hot, brush it with some of the remaining coconut oil (about 1 teaspoon) and pour two or three ¼-cup portions of batter into the pan. Cook for 2 minutes, then flip and cook for another 2 minutes, until golden brown and crispy. Transfer the pancakes to a plate and repeat with the remaining coconut oil and batter.

4. To make the coconut whipped cream, remove the canned coconut cream from the refrigerator and scoop out the solid cream portion into the chilled

mixing bowl. Using a hand mixer, mix until creamy, then add the powdered monk fruit and remaining ½ teaspoon of cinnamon. Mix again until smooth, about 2 minutes.

5. Serve the pancakes with whipped cream on top, and a little drizzle of maple syrup and sliced figs if desired.

Nutritional Analysis Per Pancake (without maple syrup and figs):
Calories: 175, Fat: 14 g, Saturated Fat: 10 g, Cholesterol: 26 mg, Fiber:
2 g, Protein: 3 g, Carbohydrates: 9 g, Sodium: 138 mg, Sugar: 1 g

Pumpkin Spice Creamer

Makes: 2½ cups
Prep time: 30 minutes plus 2 hours or overnight to soak

This delicious dairy-free creamer will take your coffee to a whole new level. A simple blend of almonds, coconut cream, and pumpkin spice comes together in a decadent but healthy creamer that will liven up your morning routine. For a quick grab-and-go snack, save the almond pulp to use in my Spiced Almond Energy Bites on page 234.

2 cups raw whole almonds
5½ cups filtered water
2 (5.4-ounce) cans coconut cream
1½ teaspoons pumpkin spice
⅛ teaspoon sea salt

1. Place the almonds in a large bowl, cover them with 3 cups of filtered water, and soak them overnight in the refrigerator. Or cover them with hot water and soak them on the countertop for 2 hours.

2. Discard the soaking water, rinse the almonds, and place them in a high-speed blender. Add the remaining 2½ cups filtered water, coconut cream, pumpkin spice, and salt. Blend for up to 2 minutes, making sure the mixture doesn't heat up.

3. Cover a mesh sieve with a nut milk bag, thin dish towel, or bandana and place over a mixing bowl. Pour in the creamer mixture and let it strain for 10 minutes.

4. After 10 minutes, gather the corners of the bag or towel and lift it up, twisting it around the almond pulp and squeezing until no more liquid comes out. Save the pulp to make my Spiced Almond Energy Bites, page 234.

5. Store the creamer in a jar or any sealed container and refrigerate for up to 5 days. Shake well and add to your favorite coffee or tea, pour over grain-free granola, or add to your favorite smoothie recipe for a warm fall-inspired flavor.

Nutritional Analysis (per 1 tablespoon): Calories: 22, Fat: 2 g, Saturated Fat: 2 g, Cholesterol: 0 mg, Fiber: 0 g, Protein: 0 g, Carbohydrates: 15 g, Sodium: 6 mg

ANTI-AGING SUPER SMOOTHIE

Serves: 1
Prep time: 5 minutes

This is one of my Master Five go-to recipes. Smoothies are a staple of my morning routine—they make it so easy to get a huge amount of phytonutrients in one glass. This one is unique in that it uses refreshing jicama, which is a great source of a soluble fiber called inulin that supports your beneficial gut bugs. Tart raspberries and pomegranate powder add a natural sweetness and tons of antioxidants for better aging.

⅓ cup jicama, peeled and cut into cubes (or unpeeled zucchini as a substitute)

½ cup fresh spinach leaves, packed

¼ cup frozen raspberries

⅓ cup coconut water

½ cup unsweetened coconut milk or other nut milk

1 tablespoon pomegranate powder

1 tablespoon nut butter (such as almond or cashew)

1 scoop grass-fed collagen powder or vanilla pumpkin seed protein powder

3 ice cubes

1. Place all the ingredients in a high-speed blender and blend until smooth.

Nutritional Analysis Per Serving (using almond butter and collagen powder): Calories: 276, Fat: 12 g, Saturated Fat: 3 g, Cholesterol: 0 mg, Fiber: 6 g, Protein: 23 g, Carbohydrates: 23 g, Sodium: 143 mg

Soups and Salads

Thai-Inspired Coconut Turkey Soup

Serves: 4
Prep time: 30 minutes
Cook time: 55 minutes

This unique spin on a Thai-style coconut soup is incredibly flavorful and satisfying. I love that it has everything I need for a nourishing meal in one bowl. For years people were afraid to enjoy dark turkey meat, but when you focus on pasture-raised high-quality turkey thighs, you get heart-healthy monounsaturated fats and immune-boosting minerals like iron, zinc, and selenium. Plus dark meat is always more tender than white meat, something every chef wants.

Turkey Balls

¾ pound pasture-raised ground turkey thighs

1 medium zucchini

1 medium carrot, peeled

1 bunch scallions

2 large garlic cloves, minced

2 tablespoons toasted sesame seeds

₋poons ground flaxseed

₋₋ salt

. pepper

₋sted sesame oil

1 pasture-raised egg

1 tablespoon coconut aminos hoisin sauce (optional)

Soup

1 tablespoon avocado oil

2 lemongrass stalks

2 shallots, peeled and thinly sliced

1 (2-inch) piece fresh ginger, peeled and thinly sliced

2 garlic cloves, peeled

4 cups low-sodium chicken broth

1 (13.5-ounce) can unsweetened full-fat coconut milk

Zest and juice of 1 lime

¼ teaspoon sea salt, plus more to taste

1 small Fresno chili, thinly sliced

1 teaspoon red curry paste

1 medium bok choy, stemmed and chopped

5 kale leaves, stemmed and chopped

1½ teaspoons gluten-free fish sauce, plus more to taste

Garnish

½ cup fresh cilantro, loosely packed

1 lime, quartered

1. Preheat the oven to 425°F.
2. Place the turkey meat in a large mixing bowl. Using the finer part of a grater, grate the zucchini and carrot into the bowl. Thinly slice the scallions, adding the white parts to the bowl and reserving the green parts.
3. Add the garlic, sesame seeds, ground flaxseed, salt, pepper, sesame oil, egg, and hoisin sauce (if using) and mix together.
4. Form and shape the turkey mixture into 2-inch balls. Place the balls on a baking dish covered with

parchment paper and bake for 20 to 25 minutes. Remove from the oven when golden brown and fragrant and set aside.

5. Meanwhile, start preparing the soup. Heat a large pot with the avocado oil over medium heat. Prepare the lemongrass by peeling off any tough outer leaves and trimming the root end. Lightly smash the stalk with the side of a knife to break it open, cut into 1-inch pieces, and add to the pot. Add the shallots and ginger. Using the wide flat side of the knife, smash the garlic and add to the pot, stirring well.

6. Cook for 5 minutes, then add the chicken broth and coconut milk. Bring the mixture to a boil, then reduce the heat to low and simmer for 35 minutes.

7. Strain the soup using a large fine-mesh strainer and add the liquids back to the pot. Add the lime zest and juice, salt, Fresno chili, red curry paste, and the baked turkey balls. Cover and continue to simmer for 10 minutes.

8. Add the bok choy and kale to the soup with the reserved green parts of the scallions, letting them wilt. Add the fish sauce, stir, and cook for 5 more minutes.

9. To serve, ladle the soup into bowls and individually garnish with cilantro and a lime wedge.

Nutritional Analysis Per Serving (without hoisin sauce): Calories: 496, Fat: 32 g, Saturated Fat: 18 g, Cholesterol: 114 mg, Fiber: 6 g, Protein: 23 g, Carbohydrates: 19 g, Sodium: 939 mg

CREAMY LEMON BASIL SOUP

Serves: 6
Prep time: 10 minutes
Cook time: 25 minutes

This is one of my Master Five go-to recipes. Fresh basil and lemon juice make this zesty soup come to life, while zucchini blends into the perfect creamy base—zero dairy needed! The combination of basil, lemon, and garlic creates potent immune support to keep you well all year long. This soup travels well, so just pour some into an insulated mug in the morning before work and you've got a hot lunch waiting.

> 1 tablespoon avocado oil
> 1 cup leeks, thinly sliced (white parts only)
> 3 large garlic cloves, roughly chopped
> 4 large zucchini, diced
> 5 cups water or low-sodium vegetable stock
> 1 teaspoon sea salt
> 10 fresh basil leaves
> ½ cup hulled hemp seeds
> ¼ cup fresh lemon juice

Garnish

> 2 tablespoons raw pine nuts
> ½ tablespoon hulled hemp seeds

1. In a medium pot, heat the avocado oil over medium-high heat. Add the leeks and sauté for 3 minutes. Add the garlic, turn the heat down to medium, and continue sautéing for 2 minutes.
2. Add the zucchini and the liquid of your choice and cover. Turn the heat down to low and simmer for 15 minutes, until the zucchini is translucent and tender.

3. Add the salt, basil, and ½ cup hemp seeds. In batches, place the soup in a high-speed blender and blend until smooth. Return to the pot, stir in the lemon juice, and bring to a boil.

4. Bring a small skillet to medium heat. Toast the pine nuts for about 2 to 3 minutes until lightly golden and fragrant. Set aside.

5. To serve, ladle the soup into bowls and garnish with hemp seeds and toasted pine nuts. Store leftovers in an airtight container in the fridge for up to 5 days.

Nutritional Analysis Per Serving (using water): Calories: 153, Fat: 11 g, Saturated Fat: 1 g, Cholesterol: 0 mg, Fiber: 3 g, Protein: 7 g, Carbohydrates: 10 g, Sodium: 385 mg

FORBIDDEN SPRING SALAD

Serves: 4
Prep time: 30 minutes
Cook time: 50 minutes

Forbidden or black rice is one of my favorite grains. Compared to white and brown rice, it's higher in protein, lower in carbs, and contains powerful antioxidants to support optimal aging and overall health. In this recipe, it's mixed with refreshing spring produce like radishes, arugula, and fresh mint for a crisp and colorful salad. Anchovies add a dose of brain-boosting omega-3 fats and a natural saltiness to the dressing.

Salad

1 cup wild black rice
2¼ cups filtered water
3 large zucchini

1 teaspoon sea salt

6 radishes

1 cup fresh mint, tightly packed

1 cup fresh parsley, tightly packed

¼ cup chives, thinly sliced

¼ medium red onion, thinly sliced

1 bunch arugula (about 3½ to 4 cups, loosely packed)

Dressing

6 anchovy fillets, marinated in olive oil, drained

¼ cup extra virgin olive oil

1 tablespoon lemon zest

2 tablespoons fresh lemon juice

2 teaspoons Dijon mustard

½ teaspoon black pepper

Garnish

½ cup raw slivered almonds

1. In a medium-size pot, combine the rice with the water and bring it to a boil. Lower the heat, cover, and let simmer for 50 minutes. Turn off the heat and leave covered for 10 more minutes. When the rice is soft but chewy, scoop into a bowl and let cool.

2. While the rice is cooking, prepare the salad. Using a mandoline or sharp knife, thinly slice the zucchini and place in a large bowl, adding the salt to help remove the water from the zucchini. Mix well and place in a colander over the sink to drain.

3. Trim the tops and ends off the radishes and cut them into quarters, roughly tear up the mint and parsley, and add all to a large mixing bowl. Add the chives, onion, and arugula to the bowl as well.

4. To make the dressing, use the back of a knife to smash the anchovy fillets and add to a small mixing bowl. Add the olive oil, lemon zest, lemon juice, mustard, and pepper and mix well.

5. In a small skillet, toast the almonds over medium heat until just golden. This should take only about 2 minutes. Set aside. Pour the drained zucchini onto a clean kitchen towel and pat dry.

6. Toss the rice, zucchini, combined vegetables and herbs, and dressing together in a large serving bowl and sprinkle the almonds over the top. Enjoy!

Nutritional Analysis Per Serving: Calories: 462, Fat: 24 g, Saturated Fat: 3 g, Cholesterol: 5 mg, Fiber: 7 g, Protein: 14 g, Carbohydrates: 53 g, Sodium: 910 mg

WASABI GINGER SPROUT SALAD

Serves: 4
Prep time: 45 minutes
Cook time: 25 minutes

This just might be the most flavorful salad you've ever had. I love the crunchy base of mung bean sprouts and shredded root vegetables combined with spicy wasabi cashews and sweet pickled ginger. If you want to prepare this ahead of time, simply leave the dressing and cashews off until you're ready to serve.

Wasabi Cashews

⅔ cup unsalted roasted cashews
1 teaspoon avocado oil
½ teaspoon wasabi powder
¼ teaspoon sea salt

Pickled Ginger

3 cups filtered water

1 (5-inch) piece fresh ginger, peeled

5 tablespoons coconut vinegar

1 tablespoon coconut sugar or granulated monk fruit

3 tablespoons beet juice or raw shredded beets

Dressing

⅓ cup avocado mayo

¼ cup coconut aminos

2 tablespoons ginger juice (from pickled ginger)

2 tablespoons finely chopped fresh cilantro

1 garlic clove, minced

¼ teaspoon sea salt

¼ teaspoon white pepper

Pinch of crushed chile flakes

Salad

2⅓ cups mung bean sprouts

1 large kohlrabi

3 large radishes

1 large jicama

½ cup chopped fresh cilantro, loosely packed

1 tablespoon black sesame seeds

1. For the wasabi cashews: Roughly chop the cashews and add them to a small bowl. Add the avocado oil, wasabi powder, and salt and mix well. Set aside.

2. Make the pickled ginger by bringing the water to a boil in a small saucepan. Using a mandoline, slice the ginger paper-thin. Once the water is boiling, add the ginger and cook for 10 minutes. Add the vinegar, sugar

or monk fruit, and beet juice or raw shredded beet to the ginger and water. Reduce the heat to medium and cook for 15 minutes. Do not drain. Set aside.

3. Make the dressing: Combine all the ingredients together in a medium jar and mix well.

4. To make the salad: Add the sprouts to a large mixing bowl. Use a mandoline to julienne the kohlrabi, radishes, and jicama. Add to the bowl along with the cilantro and black sesame seeds. Add all the pickled ginger (but discard the liquid) and toss.

5. Pour the dressing over the salad and toss gently. Sprinkle the wasabi cashews on top and serve.

Nutritional Analysis Per Serving: Calories: 497, Fat: 38 g, Saturated Fat: 6 g, Cholesterol: 30 mg, Fiber: 13 g, Protein: 8 g, Carbohydrates: 36 g, Sodium: 838 mg

CRUNCHY NAPA TEMPEH SALAD

Serves: 4
Prep time: 40 minutes
Cook time: 10 minutes

This salad has a delightful crunch from toasted almonds and snow peas, atop a refreshing, crisp mix of napa cabbage, romaine, carrots, and cucumbers. Perfectly marinated tempeh adds a little spice and a lot of savory protein. Napa cabbage is a great source of folate to support neurological and metabolic health as well as good detoxification. This salad makes an amazing one-bowl meal for lunch or dinner.

Chili Tempeh

3 tablespoons chili garlic sauce

1 tablespoon toasted sesame oil

1 (8-ounce) package gluten-free tempeh, cubed into bite-sized pieces

Napa Cabbage Salad

1 medium napa cabbage

1 large head romaine lettuce

1 medium carrot

2 Persian cucumbers

¼ large red onion

Dressing

2 tablespoons coconut vinegar or apple cider vinegar

2 tablespoons gluten-free tamari

1 tablespoon coconut aminos

1 tablespoon toasted sesame oil

¼ cup finely chopped scallions (white and green parts)

1 (½-inch) piece fresh ginger, micro-grated

Garnish

¼ cup raw sliced almonds

1 cup snow peas, strings removed, thinly sliced

¼ cup fresh cilantro or Thai basil, whole leaves, packed (optional)

2 tablespoons toasted white sesame seeds (optional)

1. Preheat the oven to 350°F and line a baking sheet with parchment paper. In a medium bowl, mix together the chili garlic sauce and toasted sesame oil. Add the tempeh cubes and set aside to marinate for 20 minutes. When ready, transfer the tempeh to the baking sheet and cook for 10 minutes.

2. To prepare the salad: Shred the cabbage and lettuce by cutting them into ½-inch strips, or use a shredder attachment on a food processor. You should have about 2 cups. Peel the carrot and cut into matchsticks to make about 1 cup. Peel and halve the cucumbers, scrape out the core, and cut into half-moons. Thinly slice the red onion and transfer all the veggies to a large bowl and toss together.

3. In a small mixing bowl, add all the dressing ingredients and mix well. Set aside.

4. Heat a small skillet over medium heat, add the almonds, and toss frequently for 3 to 5 minutes until golden and fragrant. Set aside.

5. To assemble the salad, transfer the tempeh to the bowl with the veggies, pour the dressing on top, and toss gently. Top with the almonds, snow peas, and any additional desired garnish and serve.

Nutritional Analysis Per Serving: Calories: 263, Fat: 16 g, Saturated Fat: 2 g, Cholesterol: 0 mg, Fiber: 9 g, Protein: 17 g, Carbohydrates: 20 g, Sodium: 793 mg

Entrées

SESAME-CILANTRO SALMON CAKES WITH FRESH HERB SALAD

Serves: 4 (makes 12 patties)
Prep time: 25 minutes
Cook time: 35 minutes

These savory cakes are a unique way to enjoy salmon. Topped with cilantro, mint, and basil, they're perfect for spring or summer. Salmon is an incredible source of protein and anti-inflammatory omega-3s, which benefit cognitive function, cardiovascular health, skin, and so much more.

Salmon Cakes

1 tablespoon ghee

2 large shallots, finely diced

1 stalk lemongrass, tough outer parts removed, finely chopped

1 small red bell pepper, finely diced

1 tablespoon thinly sliced red chili pepper (optional)

1 bunch scallions, finely chopped, white and green parts

3 (6-ounce) cans wild salmon, packed in olive oil, drained

½ cup chopped fresh cilantro, packed

1 tablespoon red curry paste

1 large pasture-raised whole egg

1 large pasture-raised egg white only

1 tablespoon coconut aminos

1 teaspoon toasted sesame oil

1 (1½-inch) piece fresh ginger, micro-grated

Zest of 1 lime

¼ cup ground flaxseed

¼ teaspoon curry powder

2 tablespoons toasted sesame seeds

⅛ teaspoon sea salt

Herb Salad

1 leek

1 cup fresh cilantro, loosely packed

½ cup fresh mint, loosely packed

15 fresh basil leaves (preferably Thai basil)

Dressing

1 teaspoon gluten-free low-sodium fish sauce

2 teaspoons lime juice

1 garlic clove, crushed

1 teaspoon coconut aminos

½ teaspoon toasted sesame oil

1 tablespoon yuzu sauce (optional)

1. Preheat the oven to 350°F and line a baking sheet with parchment paper.
2. Prepare the salmon cakes: Heat a medium skillet over medium heat. Add the ghee and sauté the shallots until softened, about 3 minutes. Add the lemongrass and sauté for 1 more minute. Then add the bell pepper, chili pepper (if using), and scallions and sauté for 5 minutes, stirring occasionally. Remove from the heat and set aside.
3. Add the sautéed vegetables and remaining salmon cake ingredients to a large bowl. Using your hands, mix

well and make patties about 3 inches across. Transfer to the lined sheet and bake for 10 minutes, then flip and bake for another 15 minutes until evenly browned.

4. While the patties are cooking, prepare the herb salad: Remove the green parts of the leek, and slice the white part lengthwise up the middle. Turn it over and lay it flat on the chopping board. Slice the leek into thin strips. Place in a bowl with ice water.

5. Combine the dressing ingredients in a small bowl and mix well.

6. Remove the leeks from the water, rinse well in a colander, and place on a paper towel, patting dry. Combine the leeks with the herbs in a large bowl and toss together with the dressing.

7. To serve, divide the warm patties among four plates and top with the salad. Sprinkle with more salt to taste if desired.

TRIPLE-ROASTED ROMESCO SAUCE WITH SARDINES

Serves: 4
Prep time: 30 minutes
Cook time: 45 minutes

This is one of my Master Five go-to recipes. Sardines are one of the healthiest ways to enjoy seafood. They're a low-mercury, high-omega-3 fish that supports brain health and fights inflammation. Sardines are also a really affordable way to increase your clean protein. In this recipe they're served over a super flavorful romesco sauce, made with savory roasted garlic and tangy peppers and tomatoes. Serve alongside a colorful salad or roasted veggies for a simple meal.

3 large red bell peppers

2 large Roma tomatoes

2 tablespoons avocado oil

1 whole head of garlic

¾ cup raw slivered almonds

4 scallions

4 (4¼-ounce) cans wild-caught sardines, packed in olive oil

½ teaspoon red chili flakes

¼ teaspoon black pepper

1 tablespoon sherry vinegar

½ teaspoon sea salt

¼ cup pomegranate seeds

2 tablespoons extra virgin olive oil

Pinch of Maldon or sea salt

1. Preheat the oven to 350°F. Place the whole peppers and tomatoes on a baking sheet and drizzle with the avocado oil. Wrap the head of garlic with parchment paper, then wrap with aluminum foil. Place the garlic on the baking sheet and roast in the oven for 40 minutes. Scatter the slivered almonds on the baking sheet and toast in the oven for another 5 minutes.

2. Set the tomatoes and peppers aside to cool, covered. Keep the garlic wrapped. This will help the skin separate from the flesh.

3. Meanwhile, trim off the root ends of the scallions and cut them lengthwise, julienne-style, into thin shreds. Place the scallion shreds in a bowl and cover with ice water. After 15 minutes the scallions will curl. Discard the water and transfer the scallions to a paper towel.

4. Place the sardines onto a paper towel.

5. Peel the skin from the roasted garlic, tomatoes, and peppers. Remove the seeds from the peppers, and transfer all to a food processor. Add the almonds, chili flakes, black pepper, vinegar, and ½ teaspoon sea salt. Process until smooth, about 2 minutes. Scrape the sides and process for 1 more minute.

6. Serve by spreading the sauce onto a serving plate and topping the sauce with the sardines. Garnish with the curly scallions and pomegranate seeds and drizzle with the olive oil and pinch of salt. The sauce can be saved in the refrigerator for up to a week.

Nutritional Analysis Per Serving: Calories: 511, Fat: 34 g, Saturated Fat: 5 g, Cholesterol: 43 mg, Fiber: 6 g, Protein: 36 g, Carbohydrates: 20 g, Sodium: 590 mg

LEMONY CHICKEN THIGHS WITH SUNCHOKES AND SWISS CHARD

Serves: 6
Prep time: 30 minutes
Cook time: 1 hour and 25 minutes

There's nothing like home-cooked chicken thighs for a nourishing comfort meal. In this recipe I pair them with the taste of bright lemon and sunchokes—a delicious root vegetable that acts as a beneficial prebiotic. A generous helping of Swiss chard provides immune-supporting vitamin A and bone-strengthening vitamin K.

6 bone-in, skin-on pasture-raised chicken thighs
2 tablespoons avocado oil
4 small shallots, peeled, halved lengthwise

6 large garlic cloves, peeled, thinly sliced

6 medium sunchokes, peeled, halved lengthwise or
    quartered if wide

¾ cup dry white wine (optional)

4 cups low-sodium chicken broth or water

1 small lemon, seeds removed, thinly sliced

⅓ cup fresh lemon juice

1 teaspoon fresh thyme

1 teaspoon turmeric powder

¾ teaspoon sea salt

½ teaspoon black pepper

1 bunch Swiss chard

Garnish

15 fresh mint leaves, torn

1. Place the chicken thighs on a plate and pat dry with a paper towel.

2. Place a cast-iron or heavy-bottomed skillet with a lid over medium-high heat. Add the avocado oil and, once shimmering, add the thighs skin side down. Allow them to sear, undisturbed, for about 6 minutes, until browned. Flip, and sear for another 4 minutes. Remove the thighs from the skillet and set aside.

3. Discard the oil from the pan but do not wash. To the same skillet over medium heat, add the shallots, garlic, and sunchokes. Stir for 2 minutes. Pour in the wine (if using) and allow it to reduce for 1 minute. Then add the broth or water and use a wooden spoon to scrape the bottom of the pan while heating, about 2 minutes.

4. Add the lemon slices, lemon juice, thyme, turmeric, salt, and pepper and bring to a boil. Reduce the heat to low, cover, and cook for 20 minutes.

5. After the sauce simmers for 20 minutes, nestle the thighs back into the sauce, skin side up, and braise for 25 minutes, covered.

6. Cut the chard stalks into ½-inch pieces and chop the leaves into inch-wide strips. Set aside.

7. Preheat the oven to 350°F. Once the chicken has been cooking for 25 minutes, remove the lid and add the chard, making sure the chicken is still on top.

8. Cover and transfer to the oven for 10 minutes. Then remove the lid and let the chicken brown for 10 more minutes or until it is cooked through. The skin should be extra crispy and golden.

9. To serve, place the chicken and veggies on a platter and garnish with the torn mint leaves.

Nutritional Analysis Per Serving: Calories: 321, Fat: 16 g, Saturated Fat: 3 g, Cholesterol: 75 mg, Fiber: 2 g, Protein: 26 g, Carbohydrates: 15 g, Sodium: 559 mg

EXTRA-HERBY CHICKEN-STUFFED CABBAGE

Serves: 6
Prep time: 45 minutes
Cook time: 2 hours and 30 minutes

Feed a crowd with this savory, spicy pasture-raised chicken rolled in cabbage leaves and cooked to perfection. All of the fresh herbs and spices in this recipe have loads of health benefits, like inflammation-fighting ginger and fennel, brain-boosting sage, and immuno-protective orange zest.

1 large green cabbage
4 tablespoons extra virgin olive oil

2 leeks, finely chopped

2 small fennel bulbs, finely chopped

1 bunch scallions, finely chopped

1 green serrano pepper, finely chopped

9 large garlic cloves

1½ pounds pasture-raised ground chicken

Zest of 1 large orange

1 tablespoon Szechuan peppercorns, roughly chopped

1 teaspoon ground ginger

1½ teaspoons sea salt

1 tablespoon fresh sage, minced

1 teaspoon fennel seeds

1 cup premade cauliflower rice

1 large red onion, thinly sliced

3 beef marrow bones

2 cups bone broth

½ teaspoon Chinese five-spice powder

1 tablespoon apple cider vinegar

1. Fill a large pot with enough water to cover half the cabbage and bring to a boil. Using a sharp knife, remove the toughest bottom center part of the cabbage, but try to leave the cabbage whole. Add the cabbage to the pot and boil for 10 minutes, then flip and continue boiling for another 10 minutes until tender. Discard the water and set the cabbage aside in a colander to drain.

2. While the cabbage is boiling, begin making the stuffing. Heat a large skillet with 2 tablespoons of the olive oil over medium heat. Add the leeks, fennel, scallions, and serrano pepper. Cook, stirring, for 15 minutes on medium heat until tender, then scrape into a colander and let cool.

3. Mince 3 of the garlic cloves. Add the ground chicken to the skillet over medium heat along with the minced garlic and orange zest. Cook and stir until the meat is browned, about 10 minutes. Add the Szechuan peppercorns, ginger, salt, sage, and fennel seeds and cook for 5 more minutes until all of the liquids have evaporated. Remove from the heat and stir in the cauliflower rice. Set aside to cool.

4. Place the slices of red onion in the bottom of the pot used for the cabbage and drizzle with the remaining 2 tablespoons of olive oil. Cook the onions, without stirring, for 5 minutes over medium heat. Remove from the heat.

5. Once the cabbage is dry and cooled, separate the leaves. Cut out the hard triangular rib from each cabbage leaf so that they roll easily. Scoop about ⅓ cup of stuffing onto one end of each leaf, then roll, tucking in the sides as you go.

6. Place the cabbage rolls horizontally on top of the onions, adding the marrow bones in between. Pour the bone broth on top with the remaining 6 whole garlic cloves, Chinese five-spice powder, and apple cider vinegar. Bring to a boil, then lower the heat to a low simmer, cover, and cook for 2 hours.

7. To serve, ladle cabbage rolls, onions, marrow bones, and broth into bowls and enjoy hot.

Nutritional Analysis Per Serving: Calories: 443, Fat: 23 g, Saturated Fat: 6 g, Cholesterol: 117 mg, Fiber: 10 g, Protein: 34 g, Carbohydrates: 30 g, Sodium: 853 mg

Spicy Grain-Free Steak Tacos with Olive Salsa

Serves: 6 (makes 12 tacos)
Prep time: 40 minutes
Cook time: 15 minutes

I love how the different components of a taco come together to make the perfect bite. Instead of refined corn tortillas, I make my own from grain-free cassava flour. Topped with savory grass-fed steak, grilled scallions, and a fresh herb olive salsa, these tacos are overflowing with flavor and texture. Always choose grass-fed steak for maximum nutrient density and to avoid the inflammatory fats and negative environmental effects of conventionally raised beef.

Steak and Scallions

1½ pounds grass-fed skirt steak, skin removed

1 teaspoon coarse sea salt

1 teaspoon black pepper

1 bunch scallions

3 teaspoons avocado oil

Herb Olive Salsa

½ cup finely chopped pitted green olives

1 tablespoon minced shallot

1 cup packed finely chopped fresh flat-leaf parsley

2 tablespoons finely chopped fresh oregano

1 large garlic clove, minced

1 tablespoon lemon zest (from about 1 lemon)

2 tablespoons lemon juice (from about 1 lemon)

2 tablespoons extra virgin olive oil

½ teaspoon black pepper

Cassava Tortillas

3 jalapeños, halved and seeded, finely sliced

1½ cups cassava flour

½ teaspoon sea salt

½ teaspoon garlic powder

¼ cup extra virgin olive oil

⅔ cup warm filtered water, plus more if needed

Garnish

3 limes, quartered

1. Lay the steak on a clean work surface and pat dry using a paper towel. Rub the steak with the salt and pepper. Cut the bottoms off the scallions, brush the stalks with 1 teaspoon avocado oil, and set aside. Let the steak sit at room temperature for 30 minutes before grilling while working on the salsa and tortillas.

2. Prepare the salsa by whisking together the green olives, shallots, parsley, oregano, garlic, lemon zest, lemon juice, and olive oil. Season with pepper to taste.

3. Start prepping the cassava tortillas by toasting the jalapeños in a dry pan over high heat until they start to char, about 5 minutes. Transfer to a large bowl.

4. Add the remaining tortilla ingredients to the bowl with the charred jalapeños and mix well. The dough should stick together and reach a smooth consistency. If the dough breaks, add more warm water, 1 teaspoon at a time, until it sticks together.

5. Divide the dough into 12 small balls, about the size of Ping-Pong balls. Place each ball of dough between two pieces of parchment paper and press down using a heavy pan.

6. To cook the steak: Prepare a large nonstick grill pan on high heat and add the remaining 2 teaspoons of avocado oil. Once the pan is hot, add the steak and scallions and grill for 2 minutes on each side. The steak should be well browned on the outside and still rare inside, or you can cook it longer to the desired doneness. Remove from the heat, transfer to a cutting board, and cover while finishing the tortillas.

7. Wipe the pan clean and return it to high heat. Transfer each tortilla to the hot pan, cook for 2 to 3 minutes, then flip and cook for another minute until it is lightly spotted and crisp. Transfer onto a towel, fold the towel over to cover, then repeat with the remaining dough.

8. Using a sharp knife, thinly slice the steak against the grain. Top each tortilla with steak and grilled scallions and drizzle with salsa. Serve with lime wedges.

Nutritional Analysis Per Serving: Calories: 387, Fat: 28 g, Saturated Fat: 7 g, Cholesterol: 50 mg, Fiber: 6 g, Protein: 20 g, Carbohydrates: 36 g, Sodium: 775 mg

FALL-OFF-THE-BONE SHORT RIBS WITH CASHEW "COUSCOUS"

Serves: 6
Prep time: 20 minutes
Cook time: 2 hours and 15 minutes to 2 hours and 45 minutes

The name of this recipe says it all: tender, slow-cooked ribs cooked with warm spices like cardamom and cloves are nestled alongside a nutty millet-based take on couscous. For such an impressive dish this is surprisingly easy! I love serving it for special occasions when I have a crowd to feed. Always opt for pasture-raised ribs to make sure you're eating clean, nutrient-dense meat.

Short Ribs

- 2 dried bay leaves
- 4 whole cloves
- 6 cardamom pods
- 1 teaspoon whole coriander seeds
- 4 pounds bone-in pasture-raised short ribs
- 1¼ teaspoons sea salt
- 1 teaspoon black pepper
- 1 tablespoon avocado oil
- 1 large yellow onion, finely diced
- 1 whole head of garlic, minced
- 1 (3-inch) piece fresh ginger, micro-grated
- ¼ cup apple cider vinegar
- 1 cup dry red wine
- 1 tablespoon tomato paste
- 2½ cups low-sodium vegetable stock
- 1 teaspoon paprika
- ⅛ teaspoon ground cumin
- 1 tomato, diced

Cashew "Couscous"

- ½ cup raw cashews
- 2 teaspoons avocado oil
- 1 small yellow onion, finely diced
- 1 small fennel bulb, finely diced
- 2 garlic cloves, thinly sliced
- 1 cup millet
- 2 cups low-sodium vegetable stock or filtered water
- ¼ teaspoon sea salt

½ teaspoon black pepper

½ cup loosely packed fresh flat-leaf parsley, whole leaves

1. Preheat the oven to 325°F.

2. Make a spice sachet by combining the bay leaves, whole cloves, cardamom pods, and coriander seeds and placing them into a tea bag or a coffee filter. Tie the bag with kitchen twine and set aside.

3. Dry the short ribs using a paper towel and sprinkle each side with 1 teaspoon of the salt and the pepper. In a large Dutch oven or any oven-safe heavy-bottomed pot, warm the avocado oil over medium-high heat. Once the oil is hot, place the short ribs in the pot and brown on all sides, about 45 seconds per side. Do not overcrowd the meat; sear ribs in batches.

4. Once all the ribs are nicely seared and have a good crust to them, set aside on a plate. Drain most of the oil, leaving about 2 teaspoons in the pot. Add the onion and cook over medium heat until translucent, about 5 minutes.

5. Add the garlic and ginger and cook for 30 seconds. Add the apple cider vinegar and cook for another 30 seconds until fragrant and reduced. Then add the wine and deglaze the pan using a spatula or wooden spoon, scraping the bottom well. Add the spice sachet, bring to a boil, and cook for 5 minutes until the liquid is reduced by half. Stir in the remaining ¼ teaspoon salt, tomato paste, vegetable stock, paprika, ground cumin, and diced tomato.

6. Transfer the ribs and any excess liquid back to the pot, cover, and transfer to the oven. Cook until the meat is fork-tender and falling off the bone, approximately 2

to 2½ hours, making sure to flip the meat after 1 hour. Once the meat is soft and falling off the bone, remove from the oven and allow to rest for 20 minutes with the lid on before serving.

7. After cooking the ribs for 1½ hours, prepare the couscous: Dry roast the cashews on a baking sheet in the oven for 10 minutes. Remove and set aside to cool.

8. Add the avocado oil for the couscous to a medium saucepan over medium heat. Once the oil is hot, add the onion and fennel, cook for 5 minutes until translucent, then add the garlic and cook for 2 minutes. Add the millet and stir for 1 minute, then add the vegetable stock or filtered water, salt, and pepper and bring to a boil over medium-high heat. Cover, reduce the heat to as low as possible, and simmer for 20 minutes until the liquid is absorbed. When ready, remove from the heat and set aside, covered.

9. Roughly chop the roasted cashews and sprinkle on top of the millet with the parsley. Serve the couscous warm alongside the ribs.

Nutritional Analysis Per Serving: Calories: 587, Fat: 31 g, Saturated Fat: 11 g, Cholesterol: 80 mg, Fiber: 7 g, Protein: 27 g, Carbohydrates: 42 g, Sodium: 817 mg

FARMERS' MARKET SALAD PIZZA

Serves: 4
Prep time: 35 minutes
Cook time: 50 minutes

Pizza can still be a favorite, without the dairy, gluten, and bellyache. This savory crust is made with cauliflower flour and classic Italian herbs, then it's topped with a fresh salad of arugula, heirloom tomatoes, basil, and easy pickled red onions. You can swap out the toppings for whatever is in season; some of my other favorites are spinach, peppers, and mushrooms. This is a great dish to get creative with and make your own pizza. You won't believe how good it is!

Pizza

> 2 cups cauliflower flour
> 30 fresh oregano leaves
> 1 teaspoon garlic powder
> 2 tablespoons ground flaxseed
> ¾ teaspoon sea salt
> 4 pasture-raised eggs
> 1 cup water
> 1 tablespoon avocado oil

Pickled Onions

> ½ cup red onion, thinly sliced
> 1 tablespoon sumac
> 1 tablespoon fresh lemon juice

Other Toppings

> 2 heirloom tomatoes
> ½ cup fresh basil

1 large handful arugula

2 teaspoons extra virgin olive oil

Pinch of Maldon or sea salt, or more to taste

Black pepper to taste

2 tablespoons tahini paste

1. Preheat the oven to 400°F.
2. In a medium mixing bowl, combine the cauliflower flour, oregano, garlic, flaxseed, and salt. In a separate bowl, beat the eggs with the water, then combine with the dry ingredients. Mix until a soft dough forms.
3. Line a baking sheet with parchment paper and grease with the avocado oil. Transfer the pizza dough to the center of the sheet and press down until it's ¼ inch thick. Bake in the center of the oven for 15 minutes.
4. While the crust bakes, prepare the pickled onions: Combine the thinly sliced onions with the sumac and lemon juice in a medium jar or bowl and place in the fridge until serving.
5. Prepare the other toppings: Roughly chop the tomatoes and finely chop the basil. In a large bowl, toss them together with the arugula, olive oil, Maldon salt, and pepper.
6. To assemble the pizza, top the crust evenly with the salad and pickled onions, then drizzle with the tahini. Serve immediately.

Nutritional Analysis Per Serving: Calories: 395, Fat: 18 g, Saturated Fat: 3 g, Cholesterol: 185 mg, Fiber: 13 g, Protein: 24 g, Carbohydrates: 49 g, Sodium: 738 mg

Seared Hen of the Woods Mushrooms and Smoked Porcini "Yogurt"

Serves: 4
Prep time: 15 minutes plus 30 minutes to soak
Cook time: 20 minutes

These savory mushrooms with a decadent dairy-free cream sauce make a delicious meat-free entrée. Hen of the woods mushrooms, also called maitake, are full of immune-supporting phytonutrients. They're meaty on the inside, crispy on the outside, and one of my favorite mushrooms to use in the kitchen. If you need to clean the mushrooms, don't run them under water; use a damp paper towel to wipe them and remove dirt instead.

Porcini Cashew "Yogurt"

1 cup raw cashews
½ cup dried porcini mushrooms
1 cup filtered water
Zest of 1 lemon
¼ cup fresh lemon juice
1 tablespoon extra virgin olive oil
1 large garlic clove
¼ teaspoon smoked paprika
¼ teaspoon black pepper
⅛ teaspoon sea salt

Hen of the Woods Mushrooms

3 tablespoons avocado oil
4 large garlic cloves, finely chopped
Zest from 2 lemons

4 (8-ounce) hen of the woods mushrooms, cleaned and cut in half
½ teaspoon black pepper

Garnish

2 teaspoons chopped chives
Pinch of Maldon or sea salt

1. Soak the cashews in hot water for 30 minutes. Rinse, drain, and set aside.
2. In a small saucepan, add the dried porcini mushrooms and filtered water. Bring to a boil, then reduce the heat to low and let simmer for 5 minutes. Set aside to cool.
3. Once cooled, prepare the "yogurt": Place the cashews, porcini mushrooms with water, lemon zest, lemon juice, olive oil, garlic, smoked paprika, black pepper, and sea salt in a food processor. Blend for 2 minutes until smooth, occasionally scraping the sides of the food processor. Set aside.
4. For the mushrooms: Combine 1 tablespoon avocado oil, garlic, and lemon zest in a small bowl, then set aside. Heat a heavy skillet on medium-high heat. Add the remaining 2 tablespoons avocado oil. Make sure the mushrooms are completely dry and transfer them to the skillet, cut side down, for about 2 minutes. Once they begin to soften and the edges crisp, press with a spatula to flatten.
5. Add the pepper and cook for 3 minutes per side. Reduce the heat to low, drizzle the garlic and lemon zest mixture over the top, and cook until the garlic is golden, about 1 minute. Turn the mushrooms to coat them and remove from the heat.

6. Serve by spooning the "yogurt" onto a plate and topping with the mushrooms. Garnish with the chopped chives and sprinkle with a pinch of salt.

Nutritional Analysis Per Serving: Calories: 444, Fat: 29 g, Saturated Fat: 4 g, Cholesterol: 0 mg, Fiber: 10 g, Protein: 16 g, Carbohydrates: 37 g, Sodium: 160 mg

Sides

Tangy Roasted Cauliflower

Serves: 6
Prep time: 15 minutes
Cook time: 45 minutes

Creamy tahini, tangy lemon juice, and salty capers come together to make this cauliflower ultra-flavorful. Made from sesame seeds, tahini is an excellent source of calcium. Italian parsley adds a fresh, bright finish to this tasty dish along with anti-inflammatory and antibacterial benefits. I love serving it alongside baked wild-caught salmon or roasted pasture-raised chicken thighs for a complete dinner.

1 large head cauliflower

7 large garlic cloves

1 cup tahini paste

1½ teaspoons sea salt

2 tablespoons lemon juice (from 1 medium lemon)

½ cup chopped fresh Italian parsley, loosely packed

1 cup filtered water

½ teaspoon black pepper

2 tablespoons avocado oil

2 tablespoons capers

½ cup raw sliced almonds

1. Preheat the oven to 400°F and bring a large pot of water to a boil.

2. Wash and cut the cauliflower into bite-sized florets. Add the cauliflower to the pot and boil for 5 minutes. Drain and set aside to dry.

3. To make the tahini sauce: Crush 2 garlic cloves with the flat side of a wide knife. Mix the tahini paste with the crushed garlic cloves, 1 teaspoon of the salt, lemon juice, parsley, and water until fully combined. Set aside.

4. In a large mixing bowl, season the cauliflower florets with the remaining ½ teaspoon of salt, pepper, and 1 tablespoon of avocado oil. Mix everything together until evenly coated. Transfer to a baking dish and roast for 25 minutes in the oven until tender and lightly browned.

5. Meanwhile, thinly slice the remaining 5 garlic cloves. Add the remaining 1 tablespoon of avocado oil to a small skillet with the sliced garlic and stir on medium heat for 1 minute until lightly golden. Pat the capers dry and add to the oil and garlic. Stir for 1 more minute, then remove from the heat.

6. Remove the cauliflower from the oven and pour the tahini sauce over the top, along with the oil, garlic, and caper mix.

7. Continue to bake the cauliflower for 13 minutes, then remove from the oven. Transfer to a serving platter, sprinkle the almonds on top, and allow to cool for 2 more minutes before serving.

Nutritional Analysis Per Serving: Calories: 397, Fat: 33 g, Saturated Fat: 4 g, Cholesterol: 0 mg, Fiber: 7 g, Protein: 13 g, Carbohydrates: 20 g, Sodium: 707 mg

SAUTÉED SPINACH WITH CHESTNUTS

Serves: 4
Prep time: 10 minutes
Cook time: 25 minutes

This is one of my Master Five go-to recipes. Cooked greens make a simple, nutritious, and really tasty side dish. Spinach is particularly rich in vitamin K, folate, and iron and is a superfood I suggest eating regularly. The roasted chestnuts add a slightly sweet flavor that pairs perfectly with the warm spice of freshly grated nutmeg—one of my favorite spices for supporting cognitive health.

> 3 pounds spinach
> ¼ cup avocado oil
> 1 large yellow onion, finely chopped
> 2 (5.2-ounce) bags roasted and shelled chestnuts
> ½ teaspoon freshly grated nutmeg
> ½ teaspoon white pepper
> ¾ teaspoon Maldon or sea salt

1. Wash the spinach and dry well. Chop off the stems and discard.
2. In a large pot over medium heat, add the avocado oil and onion. Sauté for 10 minutes until the onion begins to caramelize.
3. Add the spinach and sauté for 15 minutes, stirring occasionally until wilted. Meanwhile, thinly chop the chestnuts and set aside.
4. Once the spinach is wilted, season with the nutmeg, pepper, and salt and toss with the chestnuts. Serve immediately.

Nutritional Analysis Per Serving: Calories: 312, Fat: 15.4 g, Saturated Fat: 1.8 g, Cholesterol: 0 mg, Fiber: 10.6 g, Protein: 10.7 g, Carbohydrates: 39.3 g, Sodium: 638 mg

HEMP-CREAM HAZELNUT SWEET POTATOES

Serves: 6
Prep time: 20 minutes
Cook time: 40 minutes

Sweet potatoes are one of my favorite root vegetables. They're a rich source of the vitamin A precursor beta-carotene, which is essential for immune health and good eyesight, and also acts as an antioxidant. Combined with a zesty hazelnut crumb topping and fresh hemp seed cream, this is sure to be a dish the entire family will love.

Sweet Potatoes

3 long, thin sweet potatoes, unpeeled
1 tablespoon ghee
1 tablespoon smoked paprika
1¼ teaspoons sea salt
1 tablespoon black pepper

Hazelnut Crumble

1 tablespoon cumin seeds
1 tablespoon fennel seeds
1½ tablespoons ghee
½ cup blanched hazelnuts, finely chopped
¼ cup raw white sesame seeds
¼ teaspoon sea salt
Zest of 1 lemon

Hemp Seed Cream

1 cup hulled hemp seeds

1⅓ cups filtered water

2 large garlic cloves

Juice of 2 limes

2 tablespoons fresh tarragon

1 tablespoon extra virgin olive oil

½ teaspoon sea salt

1. Preheat the oven to 425°F.
2. Cut the sweet potatoes in half lengthwise. In a large mixing bowl, combine the ghee, paprika, salt, and pepper and toss with the sweet potato halves.
3. Cover a large baking sheet with parchment paper and place the sweet potatoes facedown. Bake for 30 minutes, then flip and bake for another 15 minutes.
4. To make the crumble, with a mortar and pestle grind the cumin and fennel seeds. Heat a skillet with the ghee over medium heat, adding the hazelnuts once the ghee has melted. Stir using a wooden spoon for 1 minute, then add the sesame seeds and stir for 1 minute. Add the ground cumin and fennel seeds to the skillet and stir for 2 more minutes. Then add the salt and lemon zest, stir, and remove from heat.
5. To make the hemp seed cream: Place the hemp seeds, water, garlic cloves, lime juice, tarragon, olive oil, and sea salt in a blender and blend for 2 minutes.
6. To serve, spread the hemp cream on a large plate. Place the sweet potatoes on top, then sprinkle with the hazelnut crumble.

Nutritional Analysis Per Serving: Calories: 370, Fat: 29 g, Saturated Fat: 6 g, Cholesterol: 14 mg, Fiber: 5 g, Protein: 12 g, Carbohydrates: 19 g, Sodium: 823 mg

BALSAMIC TARRAGON ROASTED ENDIVES

Serves: 4
Prep time: 5 minutes
Cook time: 5 minutes

Raw endives can be bitter, but cooking gives them a nutty, sweet flavor instead. Robust balsamic vinegar and fresh tarragon are the perfect addition to this simple yet tasty dish. Be sure to add endives to your rotation of leafy greens for some variety; they're a great source of vitamin K for bone and blood health.

4 endives
1 tablespoon ghee
2 tablespoons balsamic vinegar
¼ teaspoon sea salt
¼ teaspoon black pepper
1 tablespoon fresh tarragon

1. Cut the endives in half lengthwise.
2. Melt the ghee in a large heavy skillet over medium-high heat. Add the endives and sear for a couple of minutes per side, turning once, until golden brown but still firm in the middle.
3. Turn the heat to low, add the balsamic vinegar, salt, and black pepper, and continue to cook for 1 minute, continuously shaking the skillet to coat the endives.
4. Remove from the heat, sprinkle with the tarragon, and serve.

Nutritional Analysis Per Serving: Calories: 103, Fat: 4 g, Saturated Fat: 2 g, Cholesterol: 8 mg, Fiber: 12 g, Protein: 5 g, Carbohydrates: 14 g, Sodium: 234 mg

HOMEMADE RED LENTIL CLOUD PASTA

Serves: 6
Prep time: 30 minutes plus 45 minutes to chill and 10 minutes to rest
Cook time: 30 minutes

Pasta gets a major upgrade with this delicious dish. Red lentils are packed with protein, fiber, polyphenols, and even some iron, so they're a much healthier option than traditional pasta made from white refined flour. Lemon zest, fresh sage, and arugula give these fluffy "clouds" a bright and fresh finish; they pair perfectly as a side with roasted chicken or fish.

1½ cups dried red lentils

¾ teaspoon paprika

½ teaspoon sea salt

½ cup filtered water

3 teaspoons extra virgin olive oil

2 tablespoons ghee or coconut oil

1 tablespoon lemon zest

3 garlic cloves, thinly sliced

1½ tablespoons fresh sage, thinly sliced

½ teaspoon red chili flakes (optional)

½ teaspoon black pepper

½ teaspoon Maldon or sea salt

2 cups packed arugula

¼ cup nutritional yeast (optional)

1. Start by making lentil flour: Place the lentils in a high-speed blender and blend for 1 to 2 minutes, until a

powder forms. Using a sieve, sift the flour into a large bowl and discard the bigger chunks.

2. Place 1 cup of the lentil flour (reserve the rest for later) in a mixing bowl with the paprika and sea salt and mix together. Using your hands, create a 4-inch hole in the center. Add the water and oil into the hole, then gradually push the flour and mix into the liquid using a fork. Keep adding the flour until incorporated. The dough will be wet and sticky but should hold together as a single mass. Sprinkle in some of the leftover flour if the dough is too sticky and you are unable to form a ball. Transfer the dough to chill in the refrigerator for 45 minutes.

3. Once the dough is chilled, divide into 4 equal pieces. Dust each piece with some of the remaining lentil flour and use your hands to knead the dough, using just enough flour until the dough is no longer sticky. Roll each piece into a long skinny "snake" on your work space, approximately ½ inch in diameter (note that the dough will triple in size when cooking). Using a sharp knife, cut the "snake" into ½-inch clouds. Set aside on parchment paper and repeat with the remaining dough. Let the clouds rest, unchilled, for 10 minutes, while heating up a large pot filled with water.

4. Once the water is boiling, gently add the clouds in batches so they have room, boiling 4 minutes per batch. Scoop the clouds from the water, transfer to a sieve, and rinse with cold water. Set aside to dry. Repeat with the remaining dough.

5. When all the batches are cooked and dry, heat a large sauté pan on medium-high heat. Add the ghee. Once melted, add the lemon zest, garlic, sage, and chili flakes

(if using). Cook for 2 minutes, stirring continuously. Add the clouds and let them crisp up a bit on all sides, stirring very gently to avoid breaking them; this should take about 3 minutes. Add the black pepper, Maldon or sea salt, arugula, and nutritional yeast (if using) and serve.

Nutritional Analysis Per Serving: Calories: 235, Fat: 7 g, Saturated Fat: 3 g, Cholesterol: 11 mg, Fiber: 3 g, Protein: 12 g, Carbohydrates: 32 g, Sodium: 411 mg

SIMPLE ARRABBIATA SAUCE

Makes: 4 cups
Prep time: 10 minutes
Cook time: 45 minutes

This delicious red sauce is a must-have kitchen staple. Don't let the anchovies turn you off; they add a deeper savory, salty flavor without a fishy undertone. Cooking tomatoes actually increases the availability of powerful phytochemicals like lycopene and zeaxanthin. I love using this sauce over grain-free pasta, roasted veggies, or a crispy cauliflower pizza crust.

 2 tablespoons avocado oil
 1 (6-inch) mild green chili, cut into 1-inch cubes, or ½ teaspoon red chili flakes (optional)
 4 garlic cloves, thinly sliced
 7 anchovy fillets
 2 (28-ounce) cans whole, peeled San Marzano tomatoes
 10 Kalamata olives, pitted, quartered lengthwise
 ¾ teaspoon black pepper
 ½ cup packed fresh basil, whole leaves
 Zest of 1 lemon

1. In a large saucepan over medium-low heat, add the avocado oil, green chili or chili flakes (if using), and sliced garlic. Stir occasionally until fragrant and the peppers and garlic are lightly browned, about 7 minutes.

2. Increase the heat to medium and add the anchovy fillets, stirring and dissolving them in the hot oil for 1 minute.

3. Using your hands, squeeze the tomatoes into the pot, breaking them into large pieces. Alternately, you can roughly chop them and add them to the pot. Add the liquid from the canned tomatoes as well. Add the olives and black pepper and bring to a boil, about 2 minutes. Cover, reduce heat to medium-low, and simmer for 15 minutes to break down the tomatoes.

4. Remove the cover and, using a wooden spoon or spatula, chop up the tomatoes, stir, and let the mixture simmer for 20 minutes, stirring occasionally. Remove from the heat and stir in the basil leaves, then top with the lemon zest and serve hot.

Nutritional Analysis Per ½-Cup Serving: Calories: 100, Fat: 5 g, Saturated Fat: 1 g, Cholesterol: 3 mg, Fiber: 4 g, Protein: 3 g, Carbohydrates: 10 g, Sodium: 270 mg

Snacks

CRUNCHY WASABI-ROASTED CHICKPEAS

Serves: 6
Prep time: 30 minutes
Cook time: 40 minutes

These spicy baked chickpeas, also known as garbanzo beans, make a healthy and satisfying snack or salad topping. They're rich in protein and fiber to fill you up and couldn't be easier to make.

2 (15-ounce) cans low-sodium chickpeas
2 tablespoons avocado oil
½ teaspoon sea salt
¼ teaspoon black pepper
2 tablespoons wasabi powder
½ teaspoon garlic powder
1 teaspoon pure maple syrup (optional)

1. Drain the chickpeas in a strainer and rinse with cold water. Shake and tap the strainer, making sure to get rid of excess water. Evenly spread the chickpeas on a clean kitchen towel or paper towel and rub them dry. Let sit for at least 15 minutes, the longer the better (you can even dry them overnight).

2. Preheat the oven to 400°F. Place the chickpeas in a small mixing bowl with 1 tablespoon of avocado oil,

salt, and pepper, and evenly spread them onto a cookie sheet.

3. Transfer the cookie sheet to the oven and bake for 25 minutes. Into the same mixing bowl, add the remaining 1 tablespoon of avocado oil along with the wasabi powder and garlic powder, mix well, and set aside.

4. Remove the chickpeas from the oven and pour the wasabi mixture over the top. Stir to coat the chickpeas evenly and put them back in the oven to bake for 15 more minutes.

5. Remove the chickpeas from the oven and drizzle the maple syrup over the top, if using. Turn the oven off, but place the chickpeas back in the oven with the door cracked open for at least 10 minutes, allowing them to crisp.

6. Remove the chickpeas from the oven, allow to cool, and enjoy. I like them best fresh, but you can store them at room temperature in a sealed container for up to 5 days.

Nutritional Analysis Per Serving: Calories: 248, Fat: 9 g, Saturated Fat: 1 g, Cholesterol: 0 mg, Fiber: 10 g, Protein: 10 g, Carbohydrates: 33 g, Sodium: 205 mg

SUPERFOOD BUCKWHEAT BARS

Makes: 12 bars
Prep time: 10 minutes plus 2 hours to chill
Cook time: 5 minutes

This is one of my Master Five go-to recipes. Most energy bars at the store are loaded with artificial ingredients and refined sugar. These nourishing bars are a different story. They're packed with vitamins, minerals, longevity-boosting phyto-chemicals from wholesome buckwheat, and plenty of satiating plant-based fats and proteins from a variety of nuts, seeds, and rich cacao butter.

½ cup green buckwheat groats

⅓ cup raw Brazil nuts

½ cup unsweetened shredded coconut

⅓ cup raw sunflower seeds

⅛ teaspoon sea salt

1½ teaspoons pure vanilla extract

¼ cup raw pumpkin seeds

¼ cup whole flaxseed

¼ cup sesame seeds

¼ cup plus 1 tablespoon cacao butter

¾ cup almond butter, or any other nut butter

2 tablespoons monk fruit syrup, pure maple syrup, or raw honey

¼ cup dairy-free dark chocolate chips (preferably sweetened with monk fruit or stevia, optional)

1. In a small skillet, lightly toast the buckwheat groats over high heat, constantly shaking the pan to avoid burning. Keep shaking for 3 minutes, then remove from the heat and transfer the groats to a bowl for cooling.

2. Place the Brazil nuts, coconut, sunflower seeds, salt, and vanilla extract in a food processor. Blend for 10 seconds. Add the pumpkin seeds, whole flaxseed, and sesame seeds and process again for 10 seconds.

3. Melt all the cacao butter on low heat, using the same pan used for the buckwheat, for about 2 minutes. Add to the food processor along with the almond butter, sweetener of choice, and cooled buckwheat.

4. Process for 20 seconds. Scrape the sides using a spatula and process again for 20 seconds. The mixture should still have small chunks but also resemble a nut butter consistency. If you choose to use chocolate chips, fold them into the mix.

5. Press the mixture firmly into bar molds or an 8 x 8-inch parchment paper–lined pan. Cover and refrigerate for 2 hours.

6. If using a pan instead of molds, after chilling for 2 hours, remove the mixture from the pan and place onto a cutting board. Let sit for a couple of minutes to warm up, then cut into 12 bars.

7. Store the bars in an airtight container in the fridge for 2 weeks or in the freezer for up to 3 months.

Nutritional Analysis Per Bar: Calories: 293, Fat: 25 g, Saturated Fat: 7 g, Cholesterol: 0 mg, Fiber: 5 g, Protein: 8 g, Carbohydrates: 13 g, Sodium: 71 mg, Sugar: 1 g

SPICED ALMOND ENERGY BITES

Serves: 20
Prep time: 10 minutes
Cook time: 2 minutes

These tasty bites are the perfect pick-me-up. Even better, they use the leftover almond pulp from my Pumpkin Spice Creamer on page 187, so you don't waste a thing. The addition of spices like cinnamon and nutmeg give these the warm, satisfying taste of pumpkin pie, but with the added benefits of omega-3s from chia seeds and energy-boosting fats from shredded coconut.

6 Medjool dates, pitted

⅓ cup unsweetened shredded coconut

⅓ cup chia seeds

1 tablespoon maca powder (optional)

2 tablespoons dairy-free Pumpkin Spice Creamer (see page 187)

2 tablespoons almond butter

½ teaspoon pumpkin spice

1½ cups leftover almond pulp from Pumpkin Spice Creamer (see page 187)

1. Soak the dates in hot water for 10 minutes. In a medium pan over medium heat, toast the shredded coconut for 2 minutes until crispy and fragrant.

2. Discard the water and place the dates in a food processor along with the toasted coconut. Process until combined, then add the chia seeds, maca (if using), creamer, almond butter, and pumpkin spice. Process for 30 seconds, then add the almond pulp and process until combined.

3. Line a baking sheet with parchment paper. Using your hands, roll the mixture into 20 small balls and place, spaced apart, on the sheet.

4. Chill the bites in the freezer for 30 minutes, then enjoy. The energy bites can be stored in an airtight container in the fridge for up to 1 week or in the freezer for up to 2 months.

Nutritional Analysis Per Energy Bite: Calories: 80, Fat: 5 g, Saturated Fat: 1 g, Cholesterol: 0 mg, Fiber: 2 g, Protein: 2 g, Carbohydrates: 8 g, Sodium: 1 mg

Desserts

SNEAKY BLACK BEAN BROWNIES

Makes: 14 brownies
Prep time: 10 minutes plus 20 minutes to cool
Cook time: 25 minutes

Brownies are the perfect treat for a special occasion. These are much healthier than traditional brownies thanks to fiber-rich black beans, creamy avocado, and robust maple syrup. I promise you won't even notice the beans! And they are sure to satisfy any chocolate craving. If you prefer thicker brownies, double the ingredients, but keep in mind that changes the nutritional content.

1 (15-ounce) can low-sodium black beans

¼ avocado

1 tablespoon coconut oil, melted

2 tablespoons nut butter (preferably cashew butter)

2 teaspoons pure vanilla extract

⅓ cup ground flaxseed

1 large pasture-raised egg

⅓ cup pure maple syrup

1 tablespoon granulated monk fruit sweetener, for baking (optional)

¼ teaspoon sea salt

½ teaspoon baking powder

⅓ cup unsweetened organic cacao powder

½ cup dairy-free dark chocolate chips (preferably sweetened with monk fruit or stevia)

1. Drain the beans and rinse them well, letting them dry in a sieve. Preheat the oven to 350°F. Line an 8 x 8-inch baking dish with parchment paper.

2. Place the avocado, coconut oil, nut butter, vanilla extract, and beans in a food processor. Blend for 30 seconds until combined. Scrape the sides if needed.

3. Add the ground flaxseed, egg, maple syrup, monk fruit (if using), salt, and baking powder and process for 20 seconds.

4. Sift the cacao powder into the food processor bowl and process for 10 seconds. Scrape the sides and process for another 5 seconds. The batter should be thick and sticky.

5. Spread half of the mixture in the baking dish, sprinkle on the chocolate chips, and spread the rest of the batter on top. Smooth evenly with a spatula or the back of a spoon.

6. Place the baking dish on the top rack of the oven and bake for 25 minutes, or until the center of the brownie in the pan no longer jiggles. If testing with a toothpick, the toothpick should come out a bit sticky for fudgy brownies. Remove from the oven and let cool completely before slicing into 14 pieces. Store leftovers in an airtight container in the fridge for up to 5 days.

Nutritional Analysis Per Brownie (without monk fruit): Calories: 122, Fat: 4 g, Saturated Fat: 2 g, Cholesterol: 13 mg, Fiber: 5 g, Protein: 5 g, Carbohydrates: 17 g, Sodium: 64 mg, Sugar: 5 g

Raw Snickerdoodle Doughnuts

Makes: 20 doughnuts
Prep time: 20 minutes
Cook time: 5 minutes

I think the name of these tasty treats says it all. These cinnamon-spiced bites with a hint of vanilla and creamy coconut butter couldn't be more satisfying. They're a much healthier alternative to other sweets since they're sweetened with monk fruit, which won't cause blood sugar to spike. The healthy fats from coconut make these a satiating treat.

Doughnuts

1¼ cups almond flour
1 cup unsweetened shredded coconut
1 teaspoon pure vanilla extract
½ cup unsweetened almond milk
⅛ teaspoon sea salt
¾ teaspoon ground cinnamon
¼ cup granulated monk fruit
¼ cup coconut butter
¼ cup coconut oil

Topping

1 teaspoon cinnamon
2 tablespoons granulated monk fruit

1. Place the almond flour, shredded coconut, vanilla, almond milk, salt, cinnamon, and monk fruit in a blender.
2. In a small pan on low heat, melt the coconut butter and coconut oil.

3. Add to the blender and blend for 30 seconds until the mixture is combined into a sticky dough. Transfer the blender to the fridge and chill for 10 minutes.

4. In a small bowl, make the topping by combining the cinnamon and monk fruit. Line a sheet pan with parchment paper. Using damp hands, shape the dough into Ping-Pong-ball-sized pieces and place them on the pan. Flatten each ball slightly and sprinkle each with the cinnamon mixture.

5. Poke each doughnut with your finger to create a hole in the middle.

6. Place the doughnuts in the freezer for 10 minutes to firm up. Enjoy frozen, or refrigerated for a softer treat. Store in the freezer for up to 1 month and enjoy as a quick snack.

Nutritional Analysis (per doughnut): Calories: 114, Fat: 11 g, Saturated Fat: 6 g, Cholesterol: 0 mg, Fiber: 2 g, Protein: 2 g, Carbo-hydrates: 3 g, Sodium: 21 mg, Sugar: 1 g

EASY HONEY LAVENDER ICE CREAM

Serves: 6
Prep time: 30 minutes plus 2 hours to chill
Cook time: 8 minutes
Freeze time: 1 hour (optional, for firmer ice cream)

Lavender adds a light floral flavor and an interesting spin to this creamy dairy-free dessert. As a therapeutic herb, lavender is known for its powerful calming benefits—it reduces anxiety and promotes deeper rest and relaxation. With only 6 ingredients, this easy ice cream is just the right amount of sweet. Its unique flavor combination makes it a fun dish to serve on special occasions.

½ vanilla bean

2 (13.5-ounce) cans unsweetened full-fat coconut milk

3 tablespoons raw honey

1 tablespoon grass-fed gelatin

1½ teaspoons dried culinary lavender flowers

2 tablespoons black sesame seeds (optional)

1. Cut the vanilla bean in half lengthwise. Scrape out the seeds and combine them well with the pod, coconut milk, and honey in a medium saucepan. Add the gelatin on top and let everything sit for 5 minutes, undisturbed. Do not heat yet.

2. Mix in the gelatin and turn on the heat to low. Add the lavender flowers and whisk occasionally, cooking for a total of 8 minutes. Turn off the heat, cover, and allow the mixture to reach room temperature.

3. Once cooled, pour the mixture into a bowl through a fine sieve and refrigerate for a minimum of 2 hours or overnight.

4. Pour the refrigerated mixture into an ice cream maker and follow the manufacturer's directions for churning; this could take between 10 and 25 minutes depending on your machine. Halfway through, add the black sesame seeds, if using.

5. While the ice cream is churning, line a loaf pan with parchment paper. When the ice cream reaches the consistency of soft-serve, it can be served. For firmer ice cream, scoop it into the prepared pan, cover with plastic wrap, then freeze for 1 hour until solid.

6. If serving from the pan, let the ice cream sit out for 10 minutes at room temperature before scooping.

Nutritional Analysis Per Serving (without sesame seeds): Calories: 164, Fat: 13 g, Saturated Fat: 13 g, Cholesterol: 0 mg, Fiber: 0 g, Protein: 3 g, Carbohydrates: 11 g, Sodium: 20 mg, Sugar: 9 g

Acknowledgments

I wrote this book in hopes of putting an end to diet dogma and nutrition wars and getting more people to realize that what we all agree on is far more than we disagree on when it comes to good food and good health. We all deserve a life of vitality, and the last thing that anyone needs while healing is judgment and harsh criticism, which is pervasive these days. Revolutionizing the way we treat our bodies and the food system also requires a balanced, compassionate, and inclusive approach. This book was inspired by my patients and my community, who have expressed stress and confusion around food. I wanted to create an easy, approachable, no-nonsense guide for everyone, regardless of their dietary beliefs. This book is for you, whoever you are, and I want to say thank you. Without my community inspiring me every single day, I would not be able to show up and do the work that I do.

They say it takes a village to raise a child; well, it also takes a village to write a book. This book wouldn't have been possible without my editor, Tracy Behar, and the team at Little, Brown. I'd also like to thank my agent, Richard Pine, who has always been there for me and guided me. Of course, everyone at the Cleveland Clinic Center for

Functional Medicine and UltraWellness Center (Dr. Liz Boham, Dr. George Papanicolaou, Dr. Todd Lepine, and the entire staff) have become my functional medicine family, leading the charge to make this world a healthier place.

My message would not be as widespread without my team at Hyman Digital. I want to give a special thank-you to Courtney McNary for her beautiful illustrations and Yali Menashe and Ailsa Cowell for the delicious recipes featured in this book. I would also like to extend a huge heartfelt thanks to my business partner and captain of the ship, Dhru Purohit. To Kaya Purohit, thank you for working on this book with me and helping to spread the word that food is indeed medicine.

Finally, to my beautiful family, thank you for loving me, inspiring me, and cooking with me. Let's keep making good food together.

Resources

DR. MARK HYMAN'S WEBSITES

www.drhyman.com

For more information about the 10-Day Reset, visit getfarmacy.com.

THE ULTRAWELLNESS CENTER

55 Pittsfield Road, Suite 9

Lenox Commons

Lenox, MA 01240

If you'd like to book a virtual or in-person appointment with my clinic, visit www.ultrawellnesscenter.com or call (413) 637-9991.

BOOKS BY DR. MARK HYMAN

Food Fix

Food: What the Heck Should I Eat?

Food: What the Heck Should I Cook?

Eat Fat, Get Thin

The Eat Fat, Get Thin Cookbook

The Blood Sugar Solution 10-Day Detox Diet

The Blood Sugar Solution 10-Day Detox Diet Cookbook
The Blood Sugar Solution
The Blood Sugar Solution Cookbook
The Daniel Plan
The Daniel Plan Cookbook
UltraPrevention
UltraMetabolism
The UltraMetabolism Cookbook
The UltraSimple Diet
The UltraMind Solution

RECOMMENDED TESTS

NMR Lipid Test
www.labcorp.com

Genova Labs IgG Antibodies
www.gdx.net

Nordic Labs, DNA Diet
www.nordiclabs.com

Genetic Genie
www.geneticgenie.org

RESOURCES FOR ENDING FOOD WASTE

FreshPaper
shop.freshglow.co

Imperfect Produce
www.imperfectfoods.com

Misfits Market
www.misfitsmarket.com

SUPPLEMENT RECOMMENDATIONS

Electrolytes
BodyBio E-Lyte
www.bodybio.com

Pegan Shake Protein Powder
www.getfarmacy.com

Visit www.pegandiet.com/resources for my full list of supplement and protein powder recommendations.

ADDITIONAL RESOURCES

Environmental Working Group
www.ewg.org

Food Fix Campaign
www.foodfix.org

Clean Fish (sustainable fish)
www.cleanfish.com

A2 Milk (best milk sources)
www.a2milk.com

Community-Supported Agriculture
www.localharvest.org

Butcher Box
www.butcherbox.com

Vital Choice
www.vitalchoice.com

Thrive Market
www.thrivemarket.com

Grass Roots Meat and Poultry
www.grassrootscoop.com

KITCHEN APPLIANCES

For a full list, visit www.pegandiet.com/resources.

Vitamix Blender
www.vitamix.com

Always Pan
www.fromourplace.com

Lodge Cast-Iron Pan
www.lodgecastiron.com

Stainless Steel Pans
www.360cookware.com

Wooden Spoons and Cutting Boards
www.greenerchef.com

Thermopro Meat Thermometer
www.buythermopro.com

Notes

1 Weiss GA, Hennet T. "Mechanisms and Consequences of Intestinal Dysbiosis." *Cell Mol Life Sci.* 2017;74(16):2959–77.

2 Li Z, Henning SM, Zhang Y, et al. "Antioxidant-Rich Spice Added to Hamburger Meat During Cooking Results in Reduced Meat, Plasma, and Urine Malondialdehyde Concentrations." *Am J Clin Nutr.* 2010;91(5):1180–84.

3 Joe B, Vijaykumar M, Lokesh BR. "Biological Properties of Curcumin-Cellular and Molecular Mechanisms of Action." *Crit Rev Food Sci Nutr.* 2004;44(2):97–111.

4 Roberts CK, Barnard RJ, Sindhu RK, Jurczak M, Ehdaie A, Vaziri ND. "A High-Fat, Refined-Carbohydrate Diet Induces Endothelial Dysfunction and Oxidant/Antioxidant Imbalance and Depresses NOS Protein Expression." *J Appl Physiol (1985).* 2005;98(1):203–10.

5 Barringer TA, Hacher L, Sasser HC. "Potential Benefits on Impairment of Endothelial Function After a High-Fat Meal of 4 Weeks of Flavonoid Supplementation." *Evid Based Complement Alternat Med.* 2011;796958.

6 Neri S, Signorelli SS, Torrisi B, et al. "Effects of Antioxidant Supplementation on Postprandial Oxidative Stress and Endothelial Dysfunction: A Single-Blind, 15-Day Clinical Trial in Patients with Untreated Type 2 Diabetes, Subjects with Impaired Glucose Tolerance, and Healthy Controls." *Clin Ther.* 2005;27(11):1764–73.

7 Van Bussel BC, Henry RM, Ferreira I, et al. "A Healthy Diet Is Associated with Less Endothelial Dysfunction and Less Low-Grade Inflammation over a 7-Year Period in Adults at Risk of Cardiovascular Disease." *J Nutr.* 2015;145(3):532–40.

8 Schwingshackl L, Christoph M, Hoffmann G. "Effects of Olive Oil on Markers of Inflammation and Endothelial Function—A Systematic Review and Meta-Analysis." *Nutrients.* 2015;7(9):7651–75. Published September 11, 2015. doi:10.3390/nu7095356.

9   Gupta C, Prakash D. "Phytonutrients as Therapeutic Agents." *J Complement Integr Med.* 2014;11(3):151–69.

10 Liu M, Zhang L, Ser SL, Cumming JR, Ku KM. "Comparative Phytonutrient Analysis of Broccoli By-Products: The Potentials for Broccoli By-Product Utilization." *Molecules.* 2018;23(4):900.

11 Minich DM. "A Review of the Science of Colorful, Plant-Based Food and Practical Strategies for 'Eating the Rainbow.'" *Journal of Nutrition and Metabolism.* 2019.

12 De Souza RGM, Schincaglia RM, Pimentel GD, Mota JF. "Nuts and Human Health Outcomes: A Systematic Review." *Nutrients.* 2017; 9(12):1311.

13 Lee SA, Shu XO, Li H, et al. "Adolescent and Adult Soy Food Intake and Breast Cancer Risk: Results from the Shanghai Women's Health Study." *Am J Clin Nutr.* 2009;89(6):1920–26. doi:10.3945/ajcn.2008.27361.

14 Sytar O, Brestic M, Zivcak M, Tran LS. The Contribution of Buckwheat Genetic Resources to Health and Dietary Diversity. *Curr Genomics.* 2016;17(3):193–206. doi:10.2174/1389202917666160202215425.

15 Rowntree JE, Stanley PL, Maciel ICF, et al. 2020. "Ecosystem Impacts and Productive Capacity of a Multi-Species Pastured Livestock System." *Frontiers in Sustainable Food Systems.* In press.

16 Provenza FD, Kronberg SL, Gregorini P. "Is Grassfed Meat and Dairy Better for Human and Environmental Health?" *Front Nutr.* 2019;6:26.

17 Zeraatkar D, Han MA, Guyatt GH, et al. "Red and Processed Meat Consumption and Risk for All-Cause Mortality and Cardiometabolic Outcomes: A Systematic Review and Meta-Analysis of Cohort Studies." *Ann Intern Med.* 2019;171(10):703–10.

18 Li Z, Henning SM, Zhang Y, et al. "Antioxidant-Rich Spice Added to Hamburger Meat During Cooking Results in Reduced Meat, Plasma, and Urine Malondialdehyde Concentrations." *Am J Clin Nutr.* 2010;91(5):1180–84.

19 Willett WC, Ludwig DS. "Milk and Health." *N Engl J Med.* 2020;382(7):644–54.

20 Feskanich D, Bischoff-Ferrari HA, Frazier AL, Willett WC. "Milk Consumption During Teenage Years and Risk of Hip Fractures in Older Adults." *JAMA Pediatr.* 2014;168(1):54–60.

21 Pimpin L, Wu JH, Haskelberg H, Del Gobbo L, Mozaffarian D. "Is Butter Back? A Systematic Review and Meta-Analysis of Butter Consumption and Risk of Cardiovascular Disease, Diabetes, and Total Mortality." *PLoS One.* 2016;11(6):e0158118.

22 De Oliveira Otto MC, Lemaitre RN, Song X, King IB, Siscovick DS, Mozaffarian D. "Serial Measures of Circulating Biomarkers of Dairy Fat and Total and Cause-Specific Mortality in Older Adults: The Cardiovascular Health Study." *Am J Clin Nutr.* 2018;1–8(3):476–84.

23 "Carbon Footprint Evaluation of Regenerative Grazing at White Oak Pastures." Whiteoakpastures.com. http://blog.whiteoakpastures.com/hubfs/WOP-LCA-Quantis-2019.pdf.

24 Parker L. "A Whopping 91 Percent of Plastic Isn't Recycled." *National Geographic.* July 5, 2019.

25 Yang Q. "Gain Weight by 'Going Diet'? Artificial Sweeteners and the Neurobiology of Sugar Cravings: Neuroscience 2010." *Yale J Biol Med.* 2010;83(2):101–8.

26 Wierzejska R. "Can Coffee Consumption Lower the Risk of Alzheimer's Disease and Parkinson's Disease? A Literature Review." *Arch Med Sci.* 2017;13(3):507–14. doi:10.5114/aoms.2016.63599.

27 Dickinson A, Boyon N, Shao A. "Physicians and Nurses Use and Recommend Dietary Supplements: Report of a Survey." *Nutr J.* 2009;8:29. Published July 1, 2009. doi:10.1186/1475-2891-8-29.

28 Kang DW, Adams JB, Coleman DM, et al. "Long-Term Benefit of Microbiota Transfer Therapy on Autism Symptoms and Gut Microbiota." *Scientific Reports.* 2019;9.

29 Wang H, Lu Y, Yan Y, et al. "Promising Treatment for Type 2 Diabetes: Fecal Microbiota Transplantation Reverses Insulin Resistance and Impaired Islets." *Front Cell Infect Microbiol.* 2020;9:455.

30 Riboli E, Hunt KJ, Slimani N, et al. "European Prospective Investigation into Cancer and Nutrition (EPIC): Study Populations and Data Collection." *Public Health Nutr.* 2002;5(6B):1113–24. doi:10.1079/PHN2002394.

31 Berrazaga I, Micard V, Gueugneau M, Walrand S. "The Role of the Anabolic Properties of Plant- Versus Animal-Based Protein Sources in Supporting Muscle Mass Maintenance: A Critical Review." *Nutrients.* 2019;11(8):1825.

32 Gorissen SHM, Witard OC. "Characterising the Muscle Anabolic Potential of Dairy, Meat and Plant-Based Protein Sources in Older Adults." *Proc Nutr Soc.* 2018;77(1):20–31.

33 Jacka FN, O'Neil A, Opie R, et al. "A Randomised Controlled Trial of Dietary Improvement for Adults with Major Depression (the 'SMILES' Trial)." *BMC Med.* 2017;15:23.

34 Schoenthaler S, Amos S, Doraz W, Kelly MA, Muedeking G, Wakefield J. "The Effect of Randomized Vitamin-Mineral Supplementation

on Violent and Non-Violent Antisocial Behavior Among Incarcerated Juveniles." *J Nutr Environ Med.* January 1, 1997;7(4):343–52.

35 Rao M, Afshin A, Singh G, Mozaffarian D. "Do Healthier Foods and Diet Patterns Cost More Than Less Healthy Options? A Systematic Review and Meta-Analysis." *BMJ Open.* 2013;3(12):e004277. Published December 5, 2013. doi:10.1136/bmjopen-2013-004277.

Index

About the Author

Mark Hyman, MD, believes that we all deserve a life of vitality—and that we have the potential to create it for ourselves. That's why he is dedicated to tackling the root causes of chronic disease by harnessing the power of functional medicine to transform health care.

Dr. Hyman and his team work every day to empower people, organizations, and communities to heal their bodies and minds and to improve our social and economic resilience. Dr. Hyman is a practicing family physician, a thirteen-time #1 *New York Times* bestselling author, and an internationally recognized leader, speaker, educator, and advocate in his field. He is the head of strategy and innovation at the Cleveland Clinic Center for Functional Medicine. He is also the founder and medical director of The UltraWellness Center, chairman of the board of the Institute for Functional Medicine, and a medical editor of the *Huffington Post,* and he was a regular medical contributor on many television shows and networks, including *CBS This Morning, Today, Good Morning America,* CNN, *The View, Katie,* and *The Dr. Oz Show.* He is the host of one of the leading health podcasts, *The Doctor's Farmacy.*

Dr. Hyman works with individuals and organizations, as well as policy makers and influencers. He has testified before both the White House Commission on Complementary and Alternative Medicine and the Senate Working Group on Health Care Reform on Functional Medicine. He has consulted with the surgeon general on diabetes prevention and participated in the 2009 White House Forum on Prevention and Wellness. Senator Tom Harkin of Iowa nominated Dr. Hyman for the President's Advisory Group on Prevention, Health Promotion, and Integrative and Public Health. In addition, Dr. Hyman has worked with President Bill Clinton, presenting at the Clinton Foundation's Health Matters, Achieving Wellness in Every Generation conference, and the Clinton Global Initiative, as well as with the World Economic Forum on global health issues. He is the winner of the Linus Pauling Award, the Nantucket Project Award, and the Christian Book of the Year Award for *The Daniel Plan* and was inducted into the Books for Better Life Hall of Fame.

Dr. Hyman also works with fellow leaders in his field to help people and communities thrive. With Rick Warren, Dr. Mehmet Oz, and Dr. Daniel Amen, he created the Daniel Plan, a faith-based initiative that helped the Saddleback Church collectively lose 250,000 pounds. He is an adviser and guest co-host on *The Dr. Oz Show* and is on the board of Dr. Oz's HealthCorps, which tackles the obesity epidemic by educating American students about nutrition. With Dr. Dean Ornish and Dr. Michael Roizen, Dr. Hyman crafted and helped introduce the Take Back Your Health Act of 2009 to the United States Senate to provide for reimbursement of lifestyle treatment for chronic disease. And with Representative Tim Ryan of Ohio in 2015, he helped introduce the ENRICH Act into Congress to fund nutrition in medical education. Dr. Hyman plays a substantial role in a major film produced by Laurie David and Katie Couric, released in 2014, called *Fed Up,* which addresses childhood obesity. Please join him in helping us all take back our health at www.drhyman.com, or follow him on Twitter, Facebook, and Instagram (@drmarkhyman).